T0198203

Vaccine Hesitancy

Editors

PETER G. SZILAGYI
SHARON G. HUMISTON
TAMERA COYNE-BEASLEY

PEDIATRIC CLINICS
OF NORTH AMERICA

www.pediatric.theclinics.com

Consulting Editor
TINA L. CHENG

April 2023 • Volume 70 • Number 2

ELSEVIER

1600 John F. Kennedy Boulevard • Suite 1800 • Philadelphia, Pennsylvania, 19103-2899

http://www.theclinics.com

THE PEDIATRIC CLINICS OF NORTH AMERICA Volume 70, Number 2
April 2023 ISSN 0031-3955, ISBN-13: 978-0-443-18230-3

Editor: Kerry Holland
Developmental Editor: Axell Ivan Jade M. Purificacion

The Pediatric Clinics of North America (ISSN 0031-3955) is published bimonthly by Elsevier Inc., 360 Park Avenue South, New York, NY 10010-1710. Months of issue are February, April, June, August, October, and December. Periodicals postage paid at New York, NY and additional mailing offices. Subscription prices are $279.00 per year (US individuals), $827.00 per year (US institutions), $351.00 per year (Canadian individuals), $1100.00 per year (Canadian institutions), $419.00 per year (international individuals), $1100.00 per year (international institutions), $100.00 per year (US students and residents), $100.00 per year (Canadian students and residents), and $165.00 per year (international residents and students). To receive students/resident rare, orders must be accompanied by name of affiliated institution, date of term, and the signature of program/residency coordinator on institution letterhead. Orders will be billed at individual rate until proof of status is received. Foreign air speed delivery is included in all *Clinics* subscription prices. All prices are subject to change without notice. **POSTMASTER:** Send address changes to *The Pediatric Clinics of North America*, Elsevier Health Sciences Division, Subscription Customer Service, 3251 Riverport Lane, Maryland Heights, MO 63043. **Customer Service: 1-800-654-2452 (US and Canada). From outside of the US and Canada: 1-314-447-8871. Fax: 1-314-447-8029. For print support, E-mail: JournalsCustomerService-usa@elsevier.com. For online support, E-mail: JournalsOnlineSupport-usa@elsevier.com.**

Reprints. For copies of 100 or more, of articles in this publication, please contact the Commercial Reprints Department, Elsevier Inc., 360 Park Avenue South, New York, NY 10010-1710. Tel.: 212-633-3874; Fax: 212-633-3820; E-mail: reprints@elsevier.com.

The Pediatric Clinics of North America is also published in Spanish by McGraw-Hill Inter-americana Editores S.A., Mexico City, Mexico; in Portuguese by Riechmann and Affonso Editores, Rua Comandante Coelho 1085, CEP 21250, Rio de Janeiro, Brazil; and in Greek by Althayia SA, Athens, Greece.

The Pediatric Clinics of North America is covered in *MEDLINE/PubMed (Index Medicus), Excerpta Medica, Current Contents, Current Contents/Clinical Medicine, Science Citation Index, ASCA, ISI/BIOMED,* and *BIOSIS.*

PROGRAM OBJECTIVE
The goal of the *Pediatric Clinics of North America* is to keep practicing physicians and residents up to date with current clinical practice in pediatrics by providing timely articles reviewing the state-of-the-art in patient care.

TARGET AUDIENCE
All practicing pediatricians, physicians, and healthcare professionals who provide patient care to pediatric patients.

LEARNING OBJECTIVES
Upon completion of this activity, participants will be able to:
1. Review the topic of vaccine hesitancy in the United States.
2. Discuss vaccinations available in adolescence and young adults and the impact on prevention of severe disease.
3. Recognize how outside influences and media impact views on health and vaccination and how it can be utilized to assist in making informed decisions.

ACCREDITATIONS
Physician Credit

The Elsevier Office of Continuing Medical Education (EOCME) is accredited by the Accreditation Council for Continuing Medical Education (ACCME) to provide continuing medical education for physicians.

The EOCME designates this journal-based activity for a maximum of 13 *AMA PRA Category 1 Credit*(s)™. Physicians should claim only the credit commensurate with the extent of their participation in the activity.

All other healthcare professionals requesting continuing education credit for this journal-based activity will be issued a certificate of participation.

ABP Maintenance of Certification Credit

Successful completion of this CME activity, which includes participation in the activity and individual assessment of and feedback to the learner, enables the learner to earn up to 13 MOC points in the American Board of Pediatrics' (ABP) Maintenance of Certification (MOC) program. It is the CME activity provider's responsibility to submit learner completion information to ACCME for the purpose of granting ABP MOC credit.

DISCLOSURE OF CONFLICTS OF INTEREST
The EOCME assesses conflict of interest with its instructors, faculty, planners, and other individuals who are in a position to control the content of CME activities. All relevant conflicts of interest that are identified are thoroughly vetted by EOCME for fair balance, scientific objectivity, and patient care recommendations. EOCME is committed to providing its learners with CME activities that promote improvements or quality in healthcare and not a specific proprietary business or a commercial interest.

The planning committee, staff, authors, and editors listed below have identified no financial relationships or relationships to products or devices they or their spouse/life partner have with commercial interest related to the content of this CME activity:
Michael A. Cacciatore, PhD; James D. Campbell, MD; Pamela Gigi Chawla, MD, MHA; Tamera Coyne-Beasley, MD, MPH; Lori E. Crosby, PsyD; Jodi Cunnigham, PhD; Abigail English, JD; E. Adrianne Hammer-shaimb, MD, MS; Chad Hermann, MA; Beth L. Hoffman, PhD, MPH; Annika M. Hofstetter, MD, PhD, MPH; Lynette Jones, MSN, RN-BC; Jessica A. Kahn, MD, MPH; Joseph Kurland, MPH, CIC; Jennifer D. Kusma, MD, MS; Amisha Malhotra, MD; Rajkumar Mayakrishnan; Monica Mitchell, PhD; Daisy Y. Morales-Campos, PhD; Glen J. Nowak, PhD; Sean T. O'Leary, MD, MPH; Courtney Olson-Chen, MD, MSCI; Douglas J. Opel, MD, MPH; Cynthia M. Rand, MD, MPH; Francis J. Real, MD, MEd; Brittany L. Rosen, PhD, MEd, CHES®; Ashley B. Stephens, MD; Patricia Stinchfield, RN, MS, CPNP-PC; Melissa S. Stockwell, MD, MPH; Maria Veronica Svetaz, MD, MPH; Peter G. G. Szilagyi, MD, MPH; Leslie Walker-Harding, MD; Matthew W. Zackoff, MD, MEd

The planning committee, staff, authors, and editors listed below have identified financial relationships or relationships to products or devices they or their spouse/life partner have with commercial interest related to the content of this CME activity:
Sharon G. Humiston, MD, MPH: Consultant, Speaker: Sanofi; Researcher: GSK

Amy B. Middleman, MD, MSEd, MPH: Researcher: Pfizer, Inc.

Patricia Whitley-Williams, MD: Advisor: Merck & Co., Inc.

Todd Wolynn, MD, MMM: Consultant: Merck & Co, Inc., Sanofi Pasteur

Gregory D. Zimet, PhD: Advisor: Pfizer, Inc., Moderna, Inc.; Researcher: Merck & Co., Inc.

UNAPPROVED/OFF-LABEL USE DISCLOSURE
The EOCME requires CME faculty to disclose to the participants:
1. When products or procedures being discussed are off-label, unlabelled, experimental, and/or investigational (not US Food and Drug Administration [FDA] approved); and
2. Any limitations on the information presented, such as data that are preliminary or that represent ongoing research, interim analyses, and/or unsupported opinions. Faculty may discuss information about pharmaceutical agents that is outside of FDA-approved labelling. This information is intended solely for CME and is not intended to promote off-label use of these medications. If you have any questions, contact the medical affairs department of the manufacturer for the most recent prescribing information.

TO ENROLL
To enroll in the *Pediatric Clinics of North America* Continuing Medical Education program, call customer service at 1-800-654-2452 or sign up online at http://www.theclinics.com/home/cme. The CME program is available to subscribers for an additional annual fee of USD 324.00.

METHOD OF PARTICIPATION
In order to claim credit, participants must complete the following:
1. Complete enrolment as indicated above.
2. Read the activity.
3. Complete the CME Test and Evaluation. Participants must achieve a score of 70% on the test. All CME Tests and Evaluations must be completed online.

In order to claim MOC points, participants must complete the following:
1. Complete steps listed above for claiming CME credit
2. Provide your specialty board ID#, birth date (MM/DD), and attestation.
3. Online MOC submission is only available for the American Board of pediatrics' (ABP) Maintenance of Certification (MOC) program

CME INQUIRIES/SPECIAL NEEDS
For all CME inquiries or special needs, please contact elsevierCME@elsevier.com.

Contributors

CONSULTING EDITOR

TINA L. CHENG, MD, MPH
BK Rachford Professor and Chair of Pediatrics, University of Cincinnati, Director of the
Cincinnati Children's Research Foundation, Chief Medical Officer, Cincinnati Children's
Hospital Medical Center, Cincinnati, Ohio

EDITORS

PETER G. SZILAGYI, MD, MPH
Distinguished Professor of Pediatrics, Executive Vice-Chair and Vice-Chair for Research,
Department of Pediatrics, University of California, Los Angeles, Los Angeles, California

SHARON G. HUMISTON, MD, MPH, FAAP
Professor of Pediatrics, University of Missouri-Kansas City School of Medicine;
Department of Pediatrics, Division of Urgent Care, Children's Mercy Kansas City, Kansas
City, Missouri

TAMERA COYNE-BEASLEY, MD, MPH
Derrol Dawkins, MD Endowed Chair in Adolescent Medicine, Professor of Pediatrics and
Internal Medicine, Division Director, UAB Adolescent Medicine, Vice Chair, Pediatrics for
Community Engagement, The University of Alabama at Birmingham, Birmingham,
Alabama

AUTHORS

MICHAEL A. CACCIATORE, PhD
Associate Professor, Grady College of Journalism and Mass Communication, Co-director,
Grady Center for Health and Risk Communication, University of Georgia, Athens, Georgia

PAMELA GIGI CHAWLA, MD, MHA
Infection Preventionist, Children's Minnesota, Minneapolis, Minnesota

JAMES D. CAMPBELL, MD
Professor, Division of Infectious Diseases and Tropical Pediatrics, Department of
Pediatrics, Center for Vaccine Development and Global Health, University of Maryland
School of Medicine, Health Sciences Research Facility 1, Baltimore, Maryland

TAMERA COYNE-BEASLEY, MD, MPH
Division of Adolescent Medicine, Department of Pediatrics, The University of Alabama at
Birmingham, Birmingham, Alabama

LORI E. CROSBY, PsyD
Professor of Pediatrics, Division of Behavioral Medicine, Cincinnati Children's Hospital
Medical Center, Department of Pediatrics, University of Cincinnati College of Medicine,
Cincinnati, Ohio

JODI CUNNIGHAM, PhD
The Community Builders, Inc, Cincinnati, Ohio

ABIGAIL ENGLISH, JD
Center for Adolescent Health and the Law, Gillings School of Global Public Health, The University of North Carolina at Chapel Hill, Chapel Hill, North Carolina

E. ADRIANNE HAMMERSHAIMB, MD
Instructor, Division of Infectious Diseases and Tropical Pediatrics, Department of Pediatrics, Center for Vaccine Development and Global Health, University of Maryland School of Medicine, Health Sciences Research Facility 1, Baltimore, Maryland

CHAD HERMANN, MA
Kids Plus Pediatrics, Pittsburgh, Pennsylvania

BETH L. HOFFMAN, PhD, MPH
Department of Behavioral and Community Health Sciences, Center for Social Dynamics and Community Health, University of Pittsburgh School of Public Health, Pittsburgh, Pennsylvania

ANNIKA M. HOFSTETTER, MD, PhD, MPH
Department of Pediatrics, University of Washington School of Medicine, Seattle Children's Research Institute, M/S CURE-4, Seattle, Washington

JESSICA A. KAHN, MD, MPH
Professor, Department of Pediatrics, Cincinnati Children's Hospital Medical Center, University of Cincinnati College of Medicine, Cincinnati, Ohio

JOSEPH KURLAND, MPH, CIC
Vice President and Chief of General Pediatrics, Children's Minnesota, Minneapolis, Minnesota

JENNIFER D. KUSMA, MD, MS
Division of Advanced General Pediatrics and Primary Care, Department of Pediatrics, Ann & Robert H. Lurie Children's Hospital of Chicago, Northwestern University Feinberg School of Medicine, Chicago, Illinois

AMISHA MALHOTRA, MD
Associate Professor of Pediatrics, Division of Pediatric Allergy, Immunology and Infectious Diseases, Department of Pediatrics, Rutgers Robert Wood Johnson Medical School, New Brunswick, New Jersey

AMY B. MIDDLEMAN, MD, MSEd, MPH
OU Children's Physicians, Department of Pediatrics, University of Oklahoma Health Sciences Center, Oklahoma City, Oklahoma

MONICA MITCHELL, PhD
Professor of Pediatrics, Division of Behavioral Medicine, Department of Pediatrics, University of Cincinnati College of Medicine, Community Relations, Cincinnati Children's Hospital Medical Center, Cincinnati, Ohio

DAISY Y. MORALES-CAMPOS, PhD
Research Assistant Professor, Department of Mexican American and Latino/a Studies, Latino Research Institute, The University of Texas at Austin, Austin, Texas

GLEN J. NOWAK, PhD
Professor, Grady College of Journalism and Mass Communication, Co-director, Grady
Center for Health and Risk Communication, University of Georgia, Athens, Georgia

SEAN T. O'LEARY, MD, MPH
Professor, Department of Pediatrics, University of Colorado Anschutz Medical Campus,
Aurora, Colorado

COURTNEY OLSON-CHEN, MD, MS
Department of Obstetrics and Gynecology, University of Rochester Medical Center,
Rochester, New York

DOUGLAS J. OPEL, MD, MPH
Professor, Department of Pediatrics, University of Washington School of Medicine,
Interim Director, Treuman Katz Center for Pediatric Bioethics, Seattle Children's
Research Institute, Seattle, Washington

CYNTHIA M. RAND, MD, MPH
Department of Pediatrics, University of Rochester Medical Center, Rochester, New York

FRANCIS J. REAL, MD, MEd
Assistant Professor, Department of Pediatrics, University of Cincinnati College of
Medicine, Division of General and Community Pediatrics, Cincinnati Children's Hospital
Medical Center, Cincinnati, Ohio

BRITTANY L. ROSEN, PhD, MEd, CHES
Associate Professor, Department of Pediatrics, University of Cincinnati College of
Medicine, Division of Adolescent and Transition Medicine, Cincinnati Children's Hospital
Medical Center, Cincinnati, Ohio

ASHLEY B. STEPHENS, MD
Division of Child and Adolescent Health, Department of Pediatrics, Columbia University
Vagelos College of Physicians and Surgeons, NewYork-Presbyterian, New York, New
York

PATRICIA STINCHFIELD, RN, MS, CPNP-PC
University of Minnesota, School of Nursing, Affiliate Faculty, Pediatric Nurse Practitioner,
President, National Foundation for Infectious Diseases, Senior Director, Infection
Prevention and Control, Children's Minnesota, Minneapolis, Minnesota

MELISSA S. STOCKWELL, MD, MPH
Division of Child and Adolescent Health, Department of Pediatrics, Columbia University
Vagelos College of Physicians and Surgeons, NewYork-Presbyterian, Department of
Population and Family Health, Mailman School of Public Health, Columbia University,
New York, New York

MARIA VERONICA SVETAZ, MD, MPH
Department of Family and Community Medicine, Hennepin Healthcare, Associate
Professor, Department of Family and Community Medicine, University of Minnesota,
Minneapolis, Minnesota

LESLIE WALKER-HARDING, MD
Department of Pediatrics, Seattle Children's, Seattle, Washington

PATRICIA WHITLEY-WILLIAMS, MD
Professor of Pediatrics, Chief, Division of Pediatric Allergy, Immunology and Infectious Diseases, Department of Pediatrics, Rutgers Robert Wood Johnson Medical School, New Brunswick, New Jersey

TODD WOLYNN, MD, MMM
Kids Plus Pediatrics, Pittsburgh, Pennsylvania

MATTHEW W. ZACKOFF, MD, MEd
Assistant Professor, Department of Pediatrics, University of Cincinnati College of Medicine, Division of Critical Care Medicine, Cincinnati Children's Hospital Medical Center, Cincinnati, Ohio

GREGORY D. ZIMET, PhD
Professor of Pediatrics and Psychiatry, Department of Pediatrics, Indiana University School of Medicine, Indianapolis, Indiana

Contents

Although the term "vaccine hesitancy" has achieved great prominence, the extent to which US parents have reluctance, doubts, or indecision when it comes to vaccines recommended for children and how such hesitancy is manifest are unclear. A narrative review approach that placed emphasis on recent data and published work is used to surface evidence and insights into the current state of US parent vaccine hesitancy. The assessment finds evidence that ~6% to 25% of parents may be vaccine hesitant, that hesitancy is higher for influenza and HPV vaccines, and there are indications that addressing parent hesitancy has become more challenging.

Vaccine Hesitancy and Specific Vaccines

Although the US Advisory Committee on Immunization Practices recommends vaccinating adolescents against the human papillomavirus (HPV) to prevent HPV-associated cancers, vaccine initiation and completion rates are suboptimal. Parental and provider hesitancy contributes significantly to low HPV vaccine uptake. This review describes sources of HPV vaccine hesitancy using a World Health Organization framework that categorizes determinants of vaccine hesitancy as follows: contextual factors (historical, sociocultural, environmental, or political factors), individual and group factors (personal perception or influences of the social/peer environment), and vaccine/vaccination-specific issues (directly related to vaccine or vaccination).

Influenza vaccination rates in children are suboptimal. One underlying reason is influenza vaccine hesitancy. Tools such as the Parent Attitudes about Childhood Vaccines survey and the Vaccine Hesitancy Scale can be used to measure influenza vaccine hesitancy. The adapted Increasing Vaccination Model from Brewer and colleagues can help identify factors that influence influenza vaccine hesitancy, motivation, and uptake. Several

Early in the severe acute respiratory syndrome coronavirus 2 (SARS-CoV-2) pandemic, before coronavirus disease-2019 (COVID-19) vaccines were authorized, surveys began tracking public acceptance of a hypothetical COVID-19 vaccine. As vaccines became more widely available, the focus shifted from evaluating premeditative thoughts about COVID-19 vaccines to observing behaviors, measuring uptake, and characterizing factors associated with acceptance. A wealth of peer-reviewed literature examining the complexities of COVID-19 vaccine acceptance has emerged, but our understanding of COVID-19 vaccine acceptance is constantly evolving. In this article, we review the current state of knowledge regarding COVID-19 vaccine hesitancy, with an emphasis on pediatric vaccination.

Vaccine Hesitancy in Specific Groups

The American College of Obstetrics and Gynecology recommends influenza vaccine annually, Tdap with each pregnancy, and COVID-19 vaccine for those not previously vaccinated or who are due for boosters. The influenza and COVID-19 vaccines are safe during pregnancy and are effective in reducing morbidity in both the pregnant person and infant. The Tdap vaccine is given primarily to protect the newborn from pertussis through transplacental antibody transfer. Methods to enhance vaccination rates include stocking and giving vaccines in the obstetric office, recommending eligible vaccines at each visit, and focusing on the health of the infant in conversations with patients.

Vaccine hesitancy is an increasing global health threat, and to improve vaccine uptake, it is critical to account for identity-based considerations including racial and ethnic, religious, and contemporary socio-political identities. Using critical consciousness to create awareness of the diverse cultural viewpoints on vaccines can help providers have conversations that are identity aware, equity-focused, and linguistically sensitive with their patients. It is necessary to collaborate with patients, families, communities, and community leaders to share information about vaccines, their safety profiles, and on how to have vaccines readily accessible in each community, to protect children and adolescents against vaccine preventable illnesses.

Overcoming Parents' Vaccine Hesitancy

With more than 75% of parents and pediatric caregivers getting their health-related information online, reaching families on social media is a powerful way to leverage the trust built in the examination room to address vaccine hesitancy. This article first reviews the ways the antivaccine movement has leveraged social media to expand its considerable influence, and why social media companies have failed to reduce antivaccine misinformation and disinformation. Next, it reviews the barriers to adoption of social media-based communication by pediatric health-care providers and concludes with action-oriented items to increase the adoption of this powerful tool.

Parents trust their pediatric clinicians for up-to-date information about vaccines. To reduce vaccine hesitancy, clinics must promote confidence by building trust, communicating clearly, using patient safety and infection control principles to reduce errors, and reducing missed opportunities by having a vaccination infrastructure that makes every visit a vaccine visit. Education and communication must be consistent among all staff and culturally competent to optimize vaccine confidence. Parents have a role in seeking reliable resources, raising concerns, and seeking trusted, evidence-based experts for vaccination conversations. Safe, effective vaccines are vital; however, vaccination, a complex operational process, prevents disease and saves lives.

Vaccine acceptance by parents and caregivers remains a public health challenge that can potentially be addressed via community-based strategies. Such strategies might augment current vaccine hesitancy interventions occurring within medical homes. This article reviews the key challenges and advantages of evidence-based community strategies for overcoming parent/caregiver vaccine hesitancy, specifically (1) community-participatory vaccine hesitancy measurement, (2) communication approaches, (3) reinforcement techniques (eg, incentives, mandates), and (4) community-engaged partnerships (eg, vaccine champion training, vaccination in community settings). This article also discusses important considerations when vaccinating children and adolescents in non-primary care settings (school-based health centers, pharmacies, community events).

PEDIATRIC CLINICS OF NORTH AMERICA

Foreword

Stewardship for Science and Vaccines

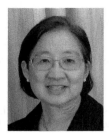

Tina L. Cheng, MD, MPH
Consulting Editor

Despite the success of vaccines in the modern world, including the rapid development of the COVID-19 vaccine, my state is now experiencing a large measles outbreak and a decline in immunization rates. At the turn of the century, the Centers for Disease Control and Prevention published "Ten Great Public Health Achievements" of the twentieth century in the United States.[1] Vaccination topped the list, a national and global success story. Other achievements included improvements in motor-vehicle safety, control of infectious diseases, safer workplaces, decline in deaths from coronary heart disease and stroke, safer and healthier foods, healthier mothers and babies, family planning, fluoridation of drinking water, and recognition of tobacco use as a health hazard.

More recently, the American Academy of Pediatrics led a campaign celebrating the Seven Great Achievements in Pediatric Research in the last 40 years.[2] Immunizations again led the list, along with reducing sudden infant death through the Back to Sleep campaign, curing a common childhood cancer, saving premature infants with surfactant, preventing HIV transmission from mother to infant, increasing life expectancy for children with chronic illnesses (eg, sickle cell disease, cystic fibrosis), and saving lives with car seats and seat belts. With the expectation of new vaccines for disease old and new, immunizations also featured prominently in prepandemic forecasts for the next great achievements in pediatric research.[3]

However, the World Health Organization listed vaccine hesitancy as one of the "Ten Threats to Global Health in 2019."[4] This prepandemic cautionary note presaged a surge in vaccine hesitancy, despite the tremendous success of the COVID-19 vaccine.

Pediatric clinicians witness the success of vaccines firsthand. I remember seeing patients with *Hemophilus influenzae* type b infection during my training. Most trainees today will not see such a patient. By building trust with children, adolescents, families,

Pediatr Clin N Am 70 (2023) xv–xvi
https://doi.org/10.1016/j.pcl.2022.12.003
0031-3955/23/© 2022 Published by Elsevier Inc.

and communities, we play a critical role in overcoming unwarranted vaccine hesitancy. Guest editors and authors in this issue lead us forward in our science-based responsibility to protect children.

Tina L. Cheng, MD, MPH
University of Cincinnati
Cincinnati Children's Research Foundation
Cincinnati Children's Hospital Medical Center
3333 Burnet Avenue MLC 3016
Cincinnati, OH 45229-3026, USA

E-mail address:
Tina.cheng@cchmc.org

REFERENCES

1. Ten Great Public Health Achievements, United States, 1900-1999. MMWR Morb Mort Wkly Rep 1999;48(12):241–3. Available at: https://www.cdc.gov/mmwr/preview/mmwrhtml/00056796.htm. Accessed December 17, 2022.
2. Cheng TL, Monteiro N, DiMeglio L, et al. Seven great achievements in pediatric research in the past 40 y. Pediatr Res 2016;80:330–7.
3. Cheng TL, Bogue CW, Dover GJ. The next 7 great achievements in pediatric research. Pediatrics 2017;139(5):e20163803.
4. World Health Organization. Ten Threats to Global Health in 2019. Available at: https://www.who.int/news-room/spotlight/ten-threats-to-global-health-in-2019. Accessed December 17, 2022.

Preface

Addressing Vaccine Hesitancy for Child and Adolescent Vaccines: The Next Big Challenge

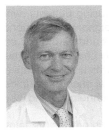 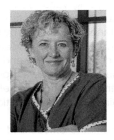 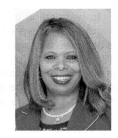

Peter G. Szilagyi, MD, MPH   Sharon G. Humiston, MD, MPH, FAAP   Tamera Coyne-Beasley, MD

Editors

When safe and effective COVID-19 vaccines were developed, it was easy to imagine that we were at the beginning of an era when everyone would recognize the stunning power of immunization to prevent illness and death from infections and to reduce societal costs. Vaccine hesitancy would be replaced by tickertape parades for everyone essential to vaccination—from the scientists who develop vaccines to the health care providers in public health, medical offices, and pharmacies who translate the scientific developments to practical protection. Antivaccine forces would lose their power as people recognized that COVID-19 vaccination saved millions of lives worldwide in the first year of use, just as smallpox, polio, measles, influenza, and pneumococcal vaccines, to specify a few, have drastically reduced morbidity and mortality from these scourges.

That, however, is not what happened. Vaccine hesitancy grew in the face of vaccine success (please see the article in this issue on the state of vaccine hesitancy in the United States). Even prior to the pandemic, the World Health Organization had designated vaccine hesitancy as one of the top 10 threats to public health, and the threat level has increased since March 2020.

This issue of *Pediatric Clinics of North America* takes a deep look at vaccine hesitancy, how it affects vaccine uptake, and what we know about strategies to address it. The articles provide an overview of vaccine hesitancy from both a public health and a clinical perspective. You will see in this issue that authors define vaccine hesitancy in different ways. However, each group of authors highlights how the factors that lead to vaccine reluctance or refusal differ depending on the vaccine (please see the articles in this issue on influenza, HPV, and COVID-19 vaccination) as well

Pediatr Clin N Am 70 (2023) xvii–xix
https://doi.org/10.1016/j.pcl.2022.12.002
0031-3955/23/© 2022 Published by Elsevier Inc.

as factors associated with the vaccination target population and decision makers. The human factors include, for example, age (please see the articles in this issue on adolescent and maternal vaccination), racial identity, culture, geography, politics, and religion. This entire journal issue, and one article in particular, emphasizes that vaccine hesitancy needs to be understood in the context of historical and contemporary racism, as well as other lived experiences, including medical exploitation, that have engendered mistrust (please see the article titled "A Structural Lens Approach to Vaccine Hesitancy and Identity").

Many authors note the important role of trust in vaccine acceptance. As trust is predicated on empathy, those of us giving vaccines are called upon to strengthen our capacity to understand the perspectives of reluctant or refusing patients, which can be a tall order when we are simultaneously drained by the poignant consequences of infectious diseases. We are being challenged by new antigens and outbreaks, such as COVID-19 and monkeypox, while confronting new and rapidly changing communication channels, such as social media and false news reports, which our patients and their families consume in large quantities prior to our brief clinical encounters (please see the articles in this issue on clinician communication, technology, and social media).

Addressing vaccine hesitancy in pediatric offices and clinics is not for the faint of heart. There is no "secret sauce" that makes interventions successful and sustainable (please see the article in this issue on optimizing your pediatric office). However, some principles seem to echo in this issue and are discussed in multiple articles. Usually more than a single-pronged approach is needed (eg, communication skills training for nursing staff and providers, including trainees, changes in practice workflow, reaching out to parents using online tools, and community-based outreach with trusted messengers). It has become clear that piling on more parent/patient education by itself is insufficient and may even be counterproductive, especially when psychological factors, including cognitive biases, are ignored.

Where do we go from here? We need a comprehensive, equity-grounded effort to address vaccine hesitancy and vaccine confidence across the lifespan. Connections between basic, social, and public health sciences must be nurtured. Partnerships must be fostered between governments, community organizations, and a wide range of sites where vaccines can be given safely (please see the article in this issue on community-based efforts). We need an infusion of fresh ideas and an exchange of cross-discipline expertise that extend far outside traditional health care. As evidence-based approaches evolve, we need to train the next generation of health care providers to do better (please see the article in this issue on training). To understand the breadth of vaccine hesitancy, a fourth C, critical consciousness, should be considered in addition to confidence, convenience, and complacency (please see article in this issue "A Structural Lens Approach to Vaccine Hesitancy and Identity"). The evolving issues related to vaccine hesitancy reflect social trends that have effects in other medical domains. What we learn from efforts to address vaccine hesitancy may be useful in these arenas, too.

A bit more than 60 years ago, an American president stood before Congress and presented a transformational challenge—to send people to the moon and bring them back safely. Today, we face a similar challenge regarding vaccine hesitancy. We need a moonshot global effort to address vaccine hesitancy even as scientific discoveries are launching new generations of vaccines. We hope this issue provides evidence to support this moonshot effort.

Peter G. Szilagyi, MD, MPH
Department of Pediatrics
University of California at Los Angeles
Los Angeles, CA 90095, USA

Sharon G. Humiston, MD, MPH, FAAP
Department of Pediatrics
Division of Urgent Care
Children's Mercy Kansas City
UMKC School of Medicine
Kansas City, MO 64106, USA

Tamera Coyne-Beasley, MD
Division of Adolescent Medicine
Department of Pediatrics
University of Alabama at Birmingham
Birmingham, AL 35233, USA

E-mail addresses:
pszilagyi@mednet.ucla.edu (P.G. Szilagyi)
sharon@immunize.org (S.G. Humiston)
tcoynebeasley@uabmc.edu (T. Coyne-Beasley)

Vaccine Hesitancy and Specific Vaccines

State of Vaccine Hesitancy in the United States

Glen J. Nowak, PhD*, Michael A. Cacciatore, PhD

KEYWORDS

- Vaccine hesitancy • Vaccine acceptance • Vaccine confidence
- Childhood vaccines

KEY POINTS

- The term "vaccine hesitancy" has achieved great prominence in recent years, but the current state of pediatric vaccine hesitancy among parents in the United States is unknown.
- It is important to undertake a regular assessment of the state of vaccine hesitancy to gauge whether and how it may be affecting parent pediatric vaccine beliefs and behaviors.
- Some findings from recent national surveys of parent compliance and intentions suggest that the current state of childhood and adolescent vaccine hesitancy in the United States is relatively stable and mostly positive.
- Other national survey findings, in concert with information from other sources, suggest a more worrisome picture of the state of parent vaccine hesitancy in the United States.
- Reluctance and unwillingness to receive recommended vaccines are significant challenges in the United States, and as such, vaccine hesitancy is a concept that rightly warrants continued attention when it comes to parent acceptance of recommended pediatric vaccines and vaccination schedules.

INTRODUCTION

A spike in measles cases in the United States in 2014 and 2015 highlighted the importance of maintaining high childhood vaccination coverage[1] and unbeknownst at the time, the beginning of much greater visibility and concern regarding the state of vaccine hesitancy. A US National Vaccine Advisory Committee (NVAC) report issued in June 2015 noted that "reluctance, hesitation, concerns, or a lack of confidence had caused some parents to question or forego recommended vaccines,"[2] and in 2019, the World Health Organization (WHO) listed "vaccine hesitancy," which they defined as "the reluctance or refusal to vaccinate despite the availability of vaccines," as one of the top threats to global health.[3] Shortly thereafter, the rapid development and availability of COVID-19 vaccines, most involving new manufacturing

Grady College of Journalism & Mass Communication, Grady Center for Health and Risk Communication, University of Georgia, 120 Hooper Street, Athens, GA 30602, USA
* Corresponding author.
E-mail address: gnowak@uga.edu

Pediatr Clin N Am 70 (2023) 197–210
https://doi.org/10.1016/j.pcl.2022.11.001
0031-3955/23/© 2022 Elsevier Inc. All rights reserved.

pediatric.theclinics.com

technologies, further increased the spotlight on vaccine hesitancy.[4,5] Although as of July 30, 2022, the US Centers for Disease Control and Prevention (CDC) reported 71% of people 5 year old and older were fully vaccinated with respect to COVID-19,[6] the vaccination recommendations continue to encounter significant and ongoing reluctance and unwillingness among the broader US adult population, including parents of children recommended to receive the vaccines.[4,7–9]

Although the term "vaccine hesitancy" has achieved great prominence,[10–12] less clear is the extent to which US parents have reluctance, doubts, or indecision when it comes to vaccines recommended for children and how such hesitancy is manifested.[13,14] Also unclear is how much vaccine hesitancy affects US parents' immunization decision-making or drives vaccine delay or refusal and in turn, childhood and adolescent vaccination uptake.[14–16] Along these lines, the 2015 NVAC report and others have endorsed efforts to regularly and systematically assess parent/caregiver beliefs, confidence, intentions, and behaviors to identify whether and how the childhood immunization landscape was changing.[2,5,11,14] Three years into a COVID-19 pandemic which has featured multiple new vaccines, disruptions in the administration of routinely recommended childhood and adolescent vaccines, and debates about COVID-19 vaccination recommendations for children,[17] assessments of the state of vaccine hesitancy in the United States with respect to routinely recommended childhood and adolescent vaccines are especially needed to sustain or achieve needed pediatric immunization uptake.[5,15,17] The assessment here does this by (1) overviewing concepts and considerations that help identify evidence or indications of vaccine hesitancy among parents and (2) using the overview as the foundation for surfacing insights into the current state of parent vaccine hesitancy in the United States. The primary focus is on infant and childhood vaccines given another article in this special issue is specifically focused on hesitancy related to adolescent vaccines (ie, those recommended for 12 to 17 year olds),[18] but pertinent findings involving parent hesitancy regarding adolescent vaccines are included.

Identifying Evidence of Vaccine Hesitancy: Key Considerations

Much recent work in the United States and across the globe has centered on conceptualizing vaccine hesitancy and identifying potential measures, signals, or indicators of hesitancy.[8,10,11,19,20] Collectively, these efforts have found that although pediatric immunization rates in the United States were (and are) generally high, vaccination uptake, delays, and declinations related to parent socio-demographics, specific vaccines, and geography exist. In addition, different definitions and measures have found vaccine hesitancy a contributing and potentially increasing barrier to pediatric vaccine uptake.[5,15] In line with this, much recent research has focused on parent hesitancy related to early childhood and adolescent COVID-19 vaccine recommendations, including to forecast COVID-19 vaccination intentions and likely uptake, inform efforts to champion COVID-19 vaccination of children, and identify any negative effects on routine childhood and adolescent vaccination confidence and uptake.[4–9,17]

Obtaining useful insights into the current state of vaccine hesitancy with respect to routinely recommended childhood and adolescent vaccines, however, is challenging. First, as published research and articles in this special issue illustrate consistent characterizations and agreed on indicators or measures of vaccine hesitancy do not exist.[19–23] Widely used early definitions, such as that from the WHO Strategic Advisory Group of Experts on Immunization (SAGE) in 2014, included behavioral as well as belief outcomes, specifically "delay or refusal of recommended vaccinations despite their availability," in the definition.[23] Such definitions, however, failed to recognize some parents who have concerns, doubts, or reluctance about vaccines fully comply with vaccination recommendations (eg, "hesitant compliers"[24] and "hesitant acceptors"[25]) or that having many questions does not mean a parent is hesitant.[9,14,19-21] These definitions also conflated hesitancy with the behavioral outcomes it is thought to cause (ie, vaccine delay or refusal) as well as diverted attention from the multiple other factors that cause parents to delay or decline recommended pediatric vaccines.[13,14,22]

More recent characterizations of vaccine hesitancy have evolved toward a focus on parents' psychological state or mindset when making immunization decisions.[14,16,19,26-29] These characterizations have encompassed degree of vaccine safety and effectiveness concerns,[9-12] "indecision" with respect to complying with a vaccination recommendation,[14,16] one's motivational state of "being conflicted or opposed to getting vaccinated,"[16,27] and beliefs, trust, and confidence regarding the importance, benefits, and risks associated with childhood and adolescent vaccines and those who endorse vaccination (eg, mainstream health care providers).[27-34] As such, a 2022 position WHO position paper on the behavioral and social drivers of vaccine uptake defined vaccine hesitancy as "a motivational state of being conflicted about, or opposed to, getting vaccinated; this includes intentions and willingness."[28] This updated definition, along with other state of mind definitions, clearly and strongly connects "hesitancy" with reluctance to receive a recommended vaccine, and in doing so, recognize that hesitancy may not result in vaccine delay or refusal of a recommended pediatric vaccine. More importantly, they provide a strong foundation for assessing the state of vaccine hesitancy in a specified group or community.[27-34] Reluctance, indecision, doubts, and presence of motivational conflict can be operationalized, measured, and validated (eg, by assessing correlations with vaccine acceptance, refusal, and delay). Further, available published studies and data can be used to find evidence and information reflective of parent vaccine-related indecision, doubts, or reluctance, including informing strategies to address hesitancy.

Two other considerations should be factored into efforts to assess a state of vaccine hesitancy, particularly if the goals include identifying its correlates and determinants, its association with pediatric vaccine uptake, or monitoring changes over time. First, although some parents' hesitancy pertains to vaccines in general, most hesitancy is "context-specific, varying across time, place, and vaccines," "influenced by factors such as complacency, convenience, and confidence" (ie, the 3 C's),[13,20-23,30,33] and associated with multiple cultural and individual-level factors, including race/ethnicity, age, and social norms.[14,20,33,34] The highly situational nature of most vaccine hesitancy means broad assessments, such as those based on national or health care practice surveys, may miss evidence of hesitancy among specific groups, in specific communities, or related to specific vaccines.[11,13,21,33,34] Also related to the state-of-mind characterizations, efforts to ascertain a state of vaccine hesitancy need to be cognizant other categories of factors influence parents' childhood and adolescent vaccination decision-making and acceptance. Thus, although doubts and concerns that foster reluctance or indecision may be real or suspected key drivers of vaccine delay or refusal, other factors could be having a greater impact.[16,21,30,34] In the 3 C's framework,[21,30] for instance, *complacency* encompasses parents' understanding of vaccine-preventable diseases (eg, the beliefs their child is susceptibility to infection or severe illness from that infection) while *convenience* centers on ease of access to affordable vaccines and patient-centered vaccination services. *Confidence* is the psychological factor that reflects trust in the safety, benefits, and effectiveness of recommended vaccines as well as those involved in vaccine licensing, manufacturing, and administration (eg, public health agencies, health care providers, and experts who formulate recommendations).[2,16,23,30-32]

Importantly, confidence and trust are two state-of-mind constructs prevalent in vaccine acceptance research and consistently found associated with vaccine hesitancy. In the "Increasing Vaccination Model" developed by Brewer and colleagues,[16,26,27] for instance, vaccine confidence, defined as "the attitude that vaccines are good (effective) or bad (unsafe)" is related to motivation to vaccinate. Parents with high confidence and trust in recommended vaccines and recommendations have higher compliance with pediatric immunization schedules, whereas those with low confidence or trust in the safety, effectiveness, or benefits of a recommended childhood or adolescent vaccine are more likely to have doubts, be reluctant to comply with a recommendation, and/or delay and decline vaccination for their child.[16,20–22,30–32] However, the 3 C's framework is also a reminder that although high levels of parent vaccine hesitancy can cause low or lower compliance with a recommended childhood or adolescent vaccine, low levels of hesitancy do not necessarily mean higher compliance with recommended vaccination schedules or high vaccine uptake.[13,16,20–22]

Approach to Assessing the State of Vaccine Hesitancy

This assessment used a narrative review approach that placed emphasis on recent data and work published within the past 5 years to surface evidence and insights into the current state of US parent vaccine hesitancy. In this assessment, we defined vaccine hesitancy as parent or caregiver doubt, indecision, or reluctance to have a child receive a recommended vaccine, which may or may not cause vaccine delay or declination. Along with this definition, the described key considerations guided the effort to find data and published articles involving US parents' actions and/or mindset regarding routinely recommended childhood and adolescent vaccines. Priority was given to data and studies related to parents actual or intended compliance with recommended childhood vaccinations, including those for adolescents, and those providing information related to parent doubts, indecision, or reluctance (ie, hesitation). Studies published since 2017 but involving data from 2016 or earlier were excluded because they were considered not well reflective of the current state of hesitancy.

The assessment begins with an overview of findings from national surveys reflective of parents' compliance and intentions with childhood vaccination schedules. The second part highlights findings related to parent vaccine decision-making, particularly beliefs and reasons parents have or hold related to doubts, indecision, and reluctance. Sources used ranged from recent CDC National Immunization Survey (NIS) results to peer-reviewed journal articles to professional commentaries and articles in respected national media outlets. It should be noted the focus here was the general state of parent vaccine hesitancy. Other articles in this special issue examine more closely human papillomavirus (HPV), influenza, and COVID-19 vaccine hesitancy, vaccine hesitancy in specific groups, and ways to address parents' vaccine hesitancy.

State of Vaccine Hesitancy: Surveys of Parent Behavior and Intentions

Despite the noted shortcomings, data and measures related to parents' actual and intended compliance with childhood and adolescent vaccination recommendations are often used to gauge the state of vaccine hesitancy.[5,11,15,20,25,29] Overall, at least three sets of insights about the current state of vaccine hesitancy among US parents can be gleaned from information in the CDCs annual NIS studies, recent assessments of childhood vaccine exemptions, and other survey results pertaining to parents' self-reported pediatric vaccination intentions and behaviors:

- *US national coverage data indicate that the vast majority of US parents are accepting of recommended childhood and adolescent vaccines.* The most recently published data from CDCs annual infant and early childhood NIS survey indicate high and/or increased uptake of recommended vaccines. Among children born in 2017 and 2018, coverage by age 24 months exceeded 90% for $\geq$3 doses of poliovirus vaccine (92.7%), $\geq$3 doses of hepatitis B (HepB) vaccine (91.9%), $\geq$1 dose of measles, mumps, and rubella vaccine (91.6%), and $\geq$1 dose of varicella vaccine (90.9).[35] There are recommended childhood vaccines for which coverage is much lower than these, but rates for almost all have been increasing. These include the full *Haemophilus* type B series (80.2%, similar to 79.8% in 2015–16); rotavirus vaccine by age 8 months (75.6% vs 73.6%), and $\geq$2 doses of influenza vaccine (60.6% vs 56%).[35] Of note, only 1.0% of children had received no vaccinations by age 24 months.[35] Also positive, recent CDC estimates of vaccination coverage nationally among kindergartners in 47 states and the District of Columbia found coverage rates of ~94% for two doses of measles, mumps, and rubella vaccine and state required doses of varicella and diphtheria, tetanus, and acellular pertussis (DTaP) vaccines.[36] This study also found the overall percentage of children with a vaccine exemption remained low during the 2020 to 21 school year (2.2%) and the percentage of children with exemptions declined in 37 states.[36] However, the study noted the COVID-19 pandemic brought multiple disruptions to vaccine administration, assessments, and tracking during the 2020 to 21 school year, with 27% of school nurses reporting that fewer students were fully vaccinated and 46% reporting that school vaccination requirements were a "somewhat lower" or "much lower" priority compared with previous years.[36] When it comes to 13 to 17 year olds, results from the 2020 NIS-Teen, the latest available and which reflect adolescent vaccination coverage before the COVID-19 pandemic, found HPV vaccination coverage ($\geq$1 dose) was 75.1% with 58.6% of teens fully up to date, whereas coverage with $\geq$1 dose of Tetanus, diphtheria, and pertussis (Tdap) and Meningococcal ACWY (MenACWY) were high and stable (90.1% and 89.3% respectively).[37] In addition, coverage surpassed 90% for $\geq$2 doses of Measles, Mumps, Rubella (MMR), $\geq$3 doses of HepB, and $\geq$1 and $\geq$ 2 doses of varicella vaccine among adolescents without a history of varicella disease.[37]

- *National coverage data provide some evidence of relatively high prevalence of hesitancy for specific vaccines (particularly influenza and HPV), some geographic regions, and certain subpopulations.* As noted above, CDC infant and early childhood NIS data collected during 2018 to 2020 found lower uptake for $\geq$4 or more doses of DTaP vaccine (81.6%), the HepB birth dose (78.4%), $\geq$2 doses of hepatitis A vaccine by 35 months (77.7%), and influenza vaccine (60.6%) relative to the other recommended vaccines.[35] Further, coverage among young children who did not have private health insurance was 9.2% to 37.8% points lower across all recommended vaccines than that for children with private insurance (except for the HepB birth dose).[35] Significant differences in vaccine uptake for many pediatric vaccines also exist across states (eg, the HepB birth dose ranged from 62.2% in Florida to 88.5% in Arizona).[35,38] This was particularly notable for influenza vaccine, where coverage among children 6 months through 17 years of age in 2020 to 21 ranged from 42.9% in Mississippi to 83.6% in Massachusetts.[39] Data from the 2020 influenza season found 59% of 5-to-12-year-old children received a flu vaccination with uptake declining to 50.8% among 13-to-17-year-old children.[37] In addition, CDCs kindergarten data found a 5% to 10% decline in MMR coverage in the 2020 to 21 school year in Maryland, Wisconsin, Georgia, Wyoming, and Kentucky,[36] whereas Zipfel and colleagues' 2020 analysis of available county-level data found that nonmedical vaccine exemptions were increasing over time in a majority of states and that several states had counties with relatively high levels of nonmedical exemptions (eg, Washington, Idaho).[40]

The 2018 to 2020 CDC NIS also shown uptake for most pediatric vaccines is lower among children of Black race or Hispanic ethnicity compared with White non-Hispanic children.[35,38] For example, the difference in influenza vaccination coverage between White children and Black children increased from 5.2% points during the 2019 to 2020 season to 11.3% points during the 2020 to 2021 season.[39]

With respect to 13 to 17 year olds, NIS-Adolescent data found that although HPV vaccination rates were ~4% points higher than in 2019, four in ten teens are partially or fully unprotected from HPV.[37] Further, a study using data from 2019 NIS-Teen classified 63% of the 13,090 parents of HPV unvaccinated adolescents as "hesitant" (ie, 8253) based on their response to the question "How likely is it that [adolescent's name] will receive HPV shots in the next 12 months?"[41] Overall, 63% were considered "very hesitant" (ie, "not at all likely), 29% were "hesitant" (ie, "somewhat unlikely), and 8% were "unsure." Non-Hispanic White parents were more often very hesitant (ie, "not at all likely") compared with Black, Hispanic, American Indian or Alaskan Native, Asian, and multiracial parents of adolescents. This is consistent with NIS-Adolescent data in recent years, which has found higher HPV vaccine coverage for Black, Hispanic, American Indian or Alaska Native, Asian, and multiracial adolescents than White adolescents (~6% to ~14% higher for ≥1 dose).[41]

- *Surveys specifically designed to obtain estimates of overall vaccine hesitancy among US parents provide some evidence of potential prevalence and correlates.* Although the COVID-19 pandemic has prompted much research into parents' intentions and hesitancy related to COVID-19 vaccines,[4,34,42] relatively few recently published studies have explicitly sought to estimate the percentage of US parents who are hesitant with respect to routinely recommended pediatric vaccines. Santibanez and colleagues included a six-item vaccine hesitancy module in the 2018 and 2019 NIS-Flu questionnaire with parents of children aged 6 to 17 months.[12] The measures in the module were developed and tested by the National Center for Health Statistics Questionnaire Design Research Laboratory[19] and focused on all recommended childhood vaccines. Key findings included: the percentage of respondents reporting they were "hesitant about childhood shots" was 25.8% in 2018% and 19.5% in 2019; hesitancy was highest for non-Hispanic Black parents (~29%); and hesitancy was inversely proportional to the child's age (ie, higher among parents of children 6–23 months). Hesitant parents had much higher concern levels regarding serious, long-term side effects (63.2% vs 11.7%) and the number of vaccines a child gets at one time (51.2% vs 11.3%) and were much less likely to have their children receive a flu vaccine (~25% point lower coverage).[12] Hesitant parents were also much more likely to indicate they personally knew someone who had a serious, long-term side effect from a vaccine (34.5% vs 8.4%).[12]

Kempe and colleagues similarly included items designed to measure vaccine hesitancy about routine and influenza vaccines in a 2019 survey of 2,176 parents/caregivers of children greater than 6 months to less than 18 year old.[43] Their survey modified a 2015 Vaccine Hesitancy Scale developed by WHOs SAGE into a scale that had eight items and four-response options for each. Hesitancy was determined by calculating the average score on the items. Key findings from their survey included: hesitancy prevalence was 6.1% for routine childhood and 25.8% for influenza vaccines; among hesitant parents, 67.5% had deferred or refused routine vaccination for their child because of concerns about that vaccine (vs 8.7% for non-hesitant parents); and an educational level lower than a bachelor's degree and household income less than 400% of the federal poverty level predicted hesitancy about both routine childhood and influenza vaccines. Race and ethnicity were not associated with hesitancy about childhood vaccines, though Hispanic parents were less hesitant about influenza vaccines than White, non-Hispanic parents.

Ellithorpe and colleagues used a self-reported behavior-focused approach to assess vaccine hesitancy in a 2019 online survey of 779 US adults who were part of an opt-in national panel.[44] Respondents had at least one child under the age of 18 and were asked to indicate if their child had ever received a vaccination and if so, whether the parent had followed the full recommended vaccination schedule for the child. This approach yielded four "childhood vaccine hesitancy groups: 53.9% who reported their child was fully vaccinated in line with the recommended schedule, 17.2% who were delayed vaccinators, 13.2% who were partial vaccinators, and 15.3% who claimed their child was "never vaccinated" (which is a percentage far higher than the ~1% found in the nationally representative CDC NIS studies and likely an artifact of the opt-in panel and inclusion of unknown number of parents of children 1 year old and younger). That said, the study found lower educational attainment (eg, high school or less) and identifying as Hispanic were associated with increased likelihood of delayed vaccination, whereas identifying as a non-Hispanic Black, lower household income, and lack of insurance were associated with increased likelihood of never vaccinating. Delayed and partial vaccinators were significantly more likely to report their child had experienced an adverse vaccine reaction such as fever, rash, or crying to a previous vaccine than complete vaccinators. Non-vaccinators were less likely than other groups to report they consulted a pediatrician about their decisions and more likely to report relying on friends and family members for vaccine information.[44]

In a study of HPV vaccine hesitancy among parents of adolescents in the United States, Szilagyi and colleagues used a 9-item Vaccine Hesitancy Scale in their national survey of 2,020 parents of adolescents 11 to 17 year old. Key findings included 23% of US parents were hesitant about HPV vaccine; most hesitant parents did not believe HPV vaccine was important for their child's health or the health of the community; hesitancy was lower among those with Hispanic, other, and multi-racial non-Hispanic ethnicity; and that overall, many parents remain concerned about HPV vaccine safety, effectiveness, and need for their adolescent.[29]

State of Vaccine Hesitancy: Evidence Related to Beliefs and Reasons

Some studies and articles in the past 5 years involving US parents and caregivers have used surveys as well as various qualitative research methods (eg, focus groups, semi-structured and unstructured interviews) to obtain insights into and understanding of vaccine hesitancy, particularly as it relates to parent beliefs involved in pediatric vaccine decision-making.[14] Along with findings from the reviewed national surveys, information from this body of research suggests three sets of insights into the state of vaccine hesitancy in the United States.

- *Many beliefs and concerns associated with parent vaccine hesitancy regarding pediatric vaccines are ones that have long been present.* Kempe and colleagues' 2019 and Santibanez and colleagues' 2018 and 2019 surveys, for instance, found vaccine hesitant parents and caregivers were highly concerned about serious side effects.[12,43] Santibanez and colleagues also found hesitancy was more prevalent among parents of children aged 6 months to 23 months (20.3%)

than parents of adolescents, with hesitancy also associated with greater concerns about the number of shots a child receives at one time.[12] Kempe and colleagues found hesitancy about influenza vaccine was driven by concerns about low vaccine effectiveness.[43] Ellithorpe and colleagues found that parents who believed their child experienced a strong or "adverse" reaction to a previous vaccine, even if the reaction was a relatively common one (eg, crying, rash, fever), were more likely to report they then used a delayed or partial vaccination strategy.[44] This is in line with Santibanez and colleagues' findings as well as those from 2012 and 2014 national parent surveys.[25] Mensah-Bonsu and colleagues' survey of parents of children with autism spectrum disorder and non-autism developmental delays found 21 of 89 were vaccine hesitant (23.6%) based on Parent Attitudes about Childhood Vaccines (PACV) scores, and these parents were more likely to believe "toxins found in vaccines/immunization" were causes of their children's delays compared with non-hesitant parents (61.9% vs 10.6%).[45]

- Parent and caregiver vaccine hesitancy also may be influenced by their moral values, faith and religious beliefs, and political identification. There is little recent published research that has systematically examined the influence of moral values, faith and religious beliefs, and political identification on parent vaccine hesitancy with respect to routinely recommended childhood vaccines but studies involving the broader US adult population suggest this worth exploring. For instance, Baumgaertner and colleagues' 2017 survey of 1006 adults from a nationally representative online panel focused on their beliefs regarding pertussis (whooping cough), measles, and influenza vaccines.[46] Their findings included: conservative-identifying respondents were less likely to indicate that they would vaccinate against pertussis, measles, and influenza than other individuals (eg, those who identified as liberals); conservative respondents tended to express lower levels of trust in institutions like the CDC than their less conservative counterparts; and respondents with lower levels of trust in government and medical experts were also less likely to express intent to vaccinate, and those individuals also tended to be conservative.[46] Similarly, studies related to COVID-19 vaccine acceptance and hesitancy involving recommendations for adults have found strong and consistent correlations with self-reported moral values (eg, liberty), faith and religious beliefs, and/or political identification.[4,8] In addition, a 2021 Religious Diversity and Vaccine Survey by the non-profit Public Religion Research Institute and Interfaith Youth Core found White Evangelicals, African-American Protestants, and Hispanic Catholics had the highest levels of COVID-19 vaccine hesitancy.[47]

With respect to moral values, Amin and colleagues found highly valuing "purity" (eg, avoiding contamination or things deemed to be unnatural) and "liberty" (eg, individual freedom) were associated with parent vaccine hesitancy.[48] In two correlational studies, medium-hesitancy parents were twice as likely as low-hesitancy parents to highly emphasize purity, and high-hesitancy respondents were twice as likely to strongly emphasize purity and liberty compared with non-hesitant parents.[48] However, the actual effects of such associations on US parents' vaccine compliance with childhood and adolescent immunization schedules remains unclear. For example, Callaghan and colleagues' 2018 on-line survey of 4,010 parents, including 2,174 who were currently parents of children under the age of 18, did not find associations between scores on a moral purity scale and self-reported delay of childhood vaccines.[49] They only found a small association with HPV vaccination hesitancy. Parents who scored highest on the moral purity scale were 8% more likely to have delayed their child's HPV vaccination than parents lowest on the scale.

- *Many parents and caregivers who are reluctant, doubtful, or indecisive seem to be more strongly questioning and/or skeptic about the value of complying with vaccine recommendations for their children.* Although strong empirical evidence involving representative samples or surveys with parents and caregivers is lacking, there are indications that many parents are more strongly questioning the need or rationale for recommended pediatric vaccines. Colgrove and Samuel's overview of "medical liberty" (ie, the belief patients have the right to choose their preferred treatment without government involvement) delineates how it is being used to present vaccine hesitancy and refusal as a civil right.[50] Descriptions of vaccine hesitancy, anti-vaccine sentiment, and parent vaccine beliefs also have been highlighted in news media articles. A May 2022 New York Times magazine article, for instance, described recent pediatrician experiences with parents whose children needed routinely recommended vaccines. Although not a study involving a representative sample of pediatricians, recurring themes from interviewed pediatricians included: frequent updates and changes in COVID-19 vaccine recommendations have reduced parent confidence in routinely recommended childhood vaccines; there seems to be an erosion of confidence in medical expertise, including more parents questioning the basis and need for routine pediatric vaccines; more parents who had previously complied with vaccination schedules are now questioning the need to follow recommended schedules (eg, booster doses); and parents who have doubts and reluctance regarding vaccines for children seem to more frequently self-characterize themselves as "pro-vaccine choice," "pro-safe vaccine," or "vaccine skeptic" rather than "anti-vaccine."[51]

DISCUSSION AND SUMMARY

As the COVID-19 pandemic has repeatedly shown, reluctance and unwillingness to receive recommended vaccines are significant challenges in the United States and as such, parent and caregiver vaccine hesitancy is a concept that rightly warrants significant and increased attention. Hesitancy may interfere with parent acceptance of recommended vaccines and vaccination schedules. As many have noted, better understanding the scope and breadth of pediatric vaccine hesitancy and the socio-demographic and other factors associated with it can strengthen vaccine education and outreach efforts and help direct resources and efforts to the primary causes of vaccination delays and low uptake.[2,5,10,15,20,43] Further, it is particularly important vaccine hesitancy reduction efforts identify and address general vaccine and medical institution mistrust among racial/ethnic communities and parents, including that related to historical and systemic racism in medicine.[34,44] However, as this assessment illustrates, the overall state of vaccine hesitancy among parents in the United States is not easy to quantify or characterize, including because systematic and significant investments in measuring and monitoring do not exist and investments in research that includes sufficient numbers of racial/ethnic groups reflective of the diversity of US parents and caregivers is lacking.[34] Rather, the broad categories of available, relatively current information and evidence reviewed here are only able to provide a suggestive limited assessment of the current state. Further, information may or may not be reflective of what is happening in most health care settings or pediatric provider practices or parent/caregiver subpopulations.

Data from recent national surveys of parent compliance and intentions suggest the current state of childhood vaccine hesitancy in the United States is broadly positive and relatively stable, though highly variable across vaccines, socio-demographic groups, geography, and pediatric provider practices. Nationally, the CDC NIS studies continue to indicate high vaccination coverage for children at ages 35 months and kindergarten entry for most recommended vaccines, whereas the percentage of children receiving no vaccines has remained at ~1%. With the exception of the first year of the COVID-19 pandemic, childhood vaccine coverage in the United States has changed little in the past 10 years.[52] CDCs immunization coverage surveys indicate much lower uptake for some vaccines, particularly influenza and HPV vaccines, some of which is due to hesitancy (ie, doubts, indecision, and reluctance) and unwillingness.[53,54] Two national surveys suggest that ~6% to ~26% of parents are vaccine hesitant with respect to routinely recommended childhood vaccines,[12,43] with more parents hesitant about influenza and HPV vaccines.[29,43] The estimated range for the former is similar to the ~19% "hesitant acceptor" and ~7% "delayer" estimates found in 2012 and 2014 national surveys,[25] whereas the higher hesitancy for influenza and HPV vaccines align with the much lower uptake rates among children.[37,39]

Other evidence from national surveys, in concert with information from health care provider reports and media stories, paints a more worrisome picture of the state of parent and caregiver vaccine hesitancy in the United States.[8,10,15,17,18,29,43] These suggest that even if uptake rates for most routinely recommended childhood vaccines are stable and quite high, or that rates have increased with respect to most vaccines where rates are lagging, troubling signs and indicators related to parent vaccine hesitancy exist. First, little progress seems to have been made addressing the long-standing beliefs and concerns that a significant number of parents continue to have regarding pediatric vaccine safety and benefits that have contributed to doubts, indecision, and reluctance. Many parents remain concerned about short-term and long-term vaccine reactions as well as the number of vaccines administered early in a child's life and/or during a single care visit. In the case of influenza, doubts about the need and value persist among many parents, and many parents remain concerned about HPV vaccine effectiveness and safety. Second, moral values and political ideologies that favor liberty, choice, and "medical freedom" seem to be more prominent factors in parent vaccine decision-making. As such, pediatricians, family physicians, and other health care professionals involved in vaccine education and administration need to be trained and equipped to address questions and concerns that go beyond vaccine safety and efficacy, such as helping parents and caregivers understand how vaccines work and the risks associated with foregoing vaccination. Also troubling are signs that political, moral, and religious considerations may be causing some parents who have previously complied with vaccine recommendations to have doubts, indecision, and reluctance[51]—which suggests education efforts have not resulted in strong and lasting understanding of the importance of pediatric vaccines and immunization schedules.

Going forward, much work remains to be done with respect to assessments of the state of parent vaccine hesitancy in the United States. The assessment here reaffirms the need for regular national, state, and practice-based studies of parent and caregiver vaccine hesitancy centered on the concepts connected to vaccine hesitancy as a psychological state. This includes measures of trust and confidence in the safety, effectiveness, and benefits of routinely recommended childhood vaccines, public health and expert recommendations and advice, and the frontline pediatricians, physicians, and health care professionals involved in vaccine education and administration. Efforts to reduce hesitancy would also benefit from studies and measures that provide better insights into the scope and basis of parent and caregiver doubts, inde-cision, and reluctance as well as help gauge the effectiveness of efforts to increase confidence and acceptance.

Reflective of the need for sound insight into parent and caregiver vaccine hesitancy, in 2021 the medical journal *The Lancet* created a Commission for Vaccine Refusal, Acceptance, and Demand in the United States to examine the state of vaccine accep-tance and formulate a public policy plan that would help increase it.[55] One facet of the Lancet Commission's undertaking is to examine "trends in vaccine hesitancy, refusal, and acceptance at the state, county, and school district levels and their effects on public health."[55] This would be a helpful examination, but these and other efforts will need to be well resourced and equipped to overcome the many challenges facing vaccine hesitancy assessments. Given that public health programs and frontline health care providers are currently dealing with significant numbers of parents and caregivers who have doubts, indecision, and reluctance regarding childhood vac-cines, well-designed and routinely implemented efforts to gauge vaccine hesitancy are well warranted and urgently needed.

CLINICS CARE POINTS

- It should be anticipated that many parents and caregivers will have reluctance, hesitancy, and doubts about recommended childhood and adolescent vaccines, including because many have relatively little knowledge regarding how vaccines provide protection or why vaccines are recommended.

- More parents likely have questions and concerns about pediatric and adolescent vaccines as a result of visible debates and persistent mis-information related to COVID-19 vaccines and vaccination recommendations.

- The state of parent and caregiver vaccine acceptance is broadly positive, but highly variable across vaccines, socio-demographic groups, geography, and pediatric provider practices.

- Regular assessments of parent and caregiver vaccine hesitancy, including efforts that have sufficient numbers of racial/ethnic reflective of the diversity of the U.S. population, are needed to strengthen vaccine acceptance and uptake.

DISCLOSURE

The authors of this article received no external funding and have no financial conflicts of interest to disclose.

REFERENCES

1. Clemmons NS, Gastanaduy PA, Fiebelkorn AP, et al. Measles — United States, January 4–April 2, 2015. Morbidity Mortality Weekly Rep 2015;64(14):373–6.
2. National Vaccine Advisory Committee. Assessing the state of vaccine confidence in the United States: recommendations from the national vaccine advisory com-mittee. Public Health Rep 2015;130:573–95.
3. World Health Organization. Top 10 threats to global health in 2019. Available at: https://www.who.int/news-room/spotlight/ten-threats-to-global-health-in-2019.
4. O'Leary S. COVID-19 vaccine hesitancy. Pediatric Clinics of North America; 2022.
5. Fisher A, Mbaeyi S, Cohn A. Addressing vaccine hesitancy in the age of COVID-19. Acad Pediatr 2021;21(4S):S3–4.

6. Centers for Disease Control and Prevention (CDC). COVID-19 Vaccinations in the United States. Available at: https://covid.cdc.gov/covid-data-tracker/# vaccinations_vacc-people-onedose-pop-5yr. Accessed July 30, 2022.

7. CDC. Estimates of vaccine hesitancy for COVID-19. Available at: https://data. cdc.gov/stories/s/Vaccine-Hesitancy-for-COVID-19/cnd2-a6zw. Accessed June 10, 2022.

8. Wang Y, Liu Y. Multilevel determinants of COVID-10 vaccination hesitancy in the United States: A rapid systematic review. Prev Med Rep 2022;25:101673.

9. Suran M. Why parents still hesitate to vaccinate their children against COVID-19. JAMA 2022;327(1):23–4.

10. Smith TC. Vaccine rejection and hesitancy: A review and call to action. Open Forum Infect Dis 2017;4(3):1–7. https://doi.org/10.1093/ofid/ofx146.

11. Salmon DA, Dudley MZ, Glanz JM, et al. Vaccine hesitancy: Causes, consequences, and a call to action. Am J Prev Med 2015;49(6S4):S391–8.

12. Santibanez TA, Nguyen KH, Greby SM, et al. Parental vaccine hesitancy and childhood influenza vaccination. Pediatrics 2020;146. e2020007609.

13. Dube E, Ward JK, Verger P, et al. Vaccine hesitancy, acceptance, and anti-vaccination: Trends and future prospects for public health. Annu Rev Public Health 2021;42:175–91.

14. Gidengil C, Chen C, Parker AM, et al. Beliefs around childhood vaccines in the United States: A systematic review. Vaccine 2019;37:6793–802.

15. Stockley S, Kempe A, Stockwell MS, et al. Improving pediatric vaccination coverage in the United States. Acad Pediatr 2021;21(4S):S1–2.

16. Brewer NT, Chapman GB, Rothman AJ, et al. Increasing vaccination: putting psychological science into action. Psychol Sci Public Interest 2017;18(3):149–207.

17. Jenssen BP, Fiks A. COVID-19 and routine childhood vaccinations- Identifying gaps and informing solutions. JAMA Pediatr 2022;176(1):21–3.

18. English A. Adolescents, young adults, and vaccine hesitancy: Who and what drives the decision to vaccinate? Pediatr Clin North America 2022.

19. Scanlon P, Jamoom E. The cognitive evaluation of survey items related to vaccine hesitance and confidence for inclusion on a series of short questions sets. Hyattsville, MD: National Center for Health Statistics; 2019.

20. Cataldi JR, O'Leary ST. Parental vaccine hesitancy: scope, causes, and potential responses. Curr Opin Infect Dis 2021;34(5):519–26.

21. MacDonald NE, Dube E, Comeau JL. Have vaccine hesitancy models oversimplified a complex problem to our detriment? The Adapted Royal Society of Canada vaccine uptake framework. Vaccine 2022. https://doi.org/10.1016/jvaccine.2022. 05.052.

22. Bedford H, Attwell K, Danchin M, et al. Vaccine hesitancy, refusal, and access barriers: the need for clarity in terminology. Vaccine 2018;36(44):6556–8.

23. MacDonald NE. Vaccine hesitancy: definition, scope and determinants. Vaccine 2015;33:4161–4.

24. Enkel SL, Attwell K, Snelling TL, et al. 'Hesitant compliers': qualitative analysis of concerned fully-vaccinating parents. Vaccine 2018;36:6459–63.

25. Chung Y, Schamel J, Fisher A, et al. Influences on immunization decision-making among U.S. parents of young children. Matern Child Health 2017;21(21): 2178–87.

26. Dudley MZ, Privor-Dumm L, Dube E, et al. Words matter: vaccine hesitancy, vaccine demand, vaccine confidence, herd immunity and mandatory vaccination. Vaccine 2020;38:709–11.

27. Brewer NT. What works to increase vaccination uptake. Acad Pediatr 2021; 21(4S):S9–15.
28. World Health Organization. Understanding the behavioural and social drivers of vaccine uptake, WHO Position Paper. Weekly Epidemiological Rec 2022; 20(97):209–24.
29. Szilagyi PG, Albertin CS, Gurfunkel D, et al. Prevalence and characteristics of HPV vaccine hesitancy among parents of adolescents across the US. Vaccine 2020;38:6027–37.
30. Betsch C, Schmid P, Heinemeier D, et al. Beyond confidence: Development of a measure assessing the 5C psychological antecedents of vaccination. PLoS One 2018;13(12):e0208601.
31. Nowak GJ, Cacciatore MA. Parents' confidence in recommended childhood vaccinations: Extending the assessment, expanding the context. Hum Vaccin Immunother 2017 Mar;13(3):687–700.
32. Gilkey MB, Magnus BE, Reiter PL, et al. The vaccination confidence scale: a brief measure of parents' vaccination beliefs. Vaccine 2014;32:6259–65.
33. Shapiro GK, Tatar O, Dube E, et al. The vaccine hesitancy scale: Psychometric properties and validation. Vaccine 2018;36:660–7.
34. Gray A, Fisher CB. Determinants of COVID-19 vaccine uptake in adolescents 12-17 years old: Examining pediatric vaccine hesitancy among racially diverse parents in the United States. Front Public Health 2022;10(3). https://doi.org/10.3389/fpubh.2022.844.310.
35. Hill HA, Yankey D, Elam-Evans LD, et al. Vaccination coverage by age 24 months children born in 2017 and 2018 – National Immunization Survey-Child, United States, 2018-2020. Morbidity Mortality Weekly Rep 2021;70(41):1435–40.
36. Seither R, Laury J, Mugerwa-Kasujj A, et al. Vaccination coverage with selected vaccines and exemption rates among children in kindergarten- United States, 2020-21. MMWR 2022;71(16):561–7.
37. Pingali C, Yankey D, Elam-Evans LD, et al. National, Regional, State, and Selected Local Area Vaccination Coverage Among Adolescents Aged 13–17 Years — United States, 2020. MMWR 2021;70(35):1183–90.
38. CDC. SUPPLEMENTARY Table 3. Vaccination Coverage by Age 24 Months Among Children Born in 2017 and 2018 — National Immunization Survey-Child, United States, 2018–2020. Available at: https://stacks.cdc.gov/view/cdc/110377. Accessed June 18, 2022.
39. CDC. Flu Vaccination Coverage, United States, 2020–21 Influenza Season. Available at: https://www.cdc.gov/flu/fluvaxview/coverage-2021estimates.htm. Accessed June 14, 2022.
40. Zipfel CM, Garnier R, Kuney MC, et al. The landscape of childhood vaccine exemptions in the United States 2020. Scientific Data;7(401). https://doi.org/10.1038/s41597-020-00742-5
41. Rositch AF, Liu T, Chao C, et al. Levels of parental Human Papillomavirus vaccine hesitancy and their reasons for not intending to vaccinate: Insights from the 2019 NIS-Teen. J Adolesc Health 2022;71:39–46.
42. Ellithorpe ME, Aladé F, Adams RB, et al. Looking ahead: Caregivers' COVID-19 vaccination intention for children 5 years old and younger using the health belief model. Vaccine 2022;40(10):1404–12.
43. Kempe A, Saville AW, Albertin C, et al. Parental hesitancy about routine childhood and influenza vaccinations: a national survey. Pediatrics 2020;146(1):e20193852.

44. Ellithorpe ME, Adams R, Alade F. Parents' behaviors and experiences associated with four vaccination behavior groups for childhood vaccine hesitancy. Matern Child Health J 2022;26:280–8.

45. Mensah-Bonsu NE, Mire SS, Sahni LC, et al. Understanding vaccine hesitancy among parents of children with Autism Spectrum Disorder and Parents of Children with non-Autism Developmental Delays. J Child Neurol 2021;36(10):911–8.

46. Baumgaertner B, Carlisle JE, Justwan F. The influence of political ideology and trust on willingness to vaccinate. PLoS ONE 2018;13(1):e0191728.

47. Public Religious Research Institute & the Interfaith Youth Core. Religious Diversity and Vaccine Survey 2021. Available at: https://www.prri.org/research/religious-identities-and-the-race-against-the-virus-american-attitudes-on-vaccination-mandates-and-religious-exemptions/. Accessed June 20, 2022.

48. Amin A, Bednarczyk RA, Ray CE, et al. Association of moral values with vaccine hesitancy. Nat Hum Behav 2017;1(12):873–80.

49. Callaghan T, Motta M, Sylvester S, et al. Parent psychology and the decision to delay childhood vaccination. Social Sci Med 2019;238(112407):1–8.

50. Colgrove J, Samuel SJ. Freedom, rights, and vaccine refusal: The history of an idea. Am J Public Health 2022;112(2):234–41.

51. Velasquez-Manoff M. The anti-vaccine movement's new frontier. New York: New York Times Magazine; 2022.

52. CDC. NIS-Child Vaccination Coverage Reports. Available at: https://www.cdc.gov/vaccines/imz-managers/coverage/childvaxview/pubs-presentations.html. Accessed June 20, 2022.

53. Stockwell M. Influenza vaccine hesitancy. Pediatric Clinics of North America; 2022.

54. Morales-Campos D. HPV vaccine hesitancy. Pediatric Clinics of North America; 2022.

55. Commissioners of the *Lancet* Commission on Vaccine Refusal, Acceptance, and Demand for the USA. Announcing the *Lancet* Commission on Vaccine Refusal, Acceptance, and Demand in the USA. Lancet 2021;3:21.

Human Papillomavirus Vaccine Hesitancy in the United States

Daisy Y. Morales-Campos, PhD[a],*, Gregory D. Zimet, PhD[b],
Jessica A. Kahn, MD, MPH[c]

KEYWORDS

- Adolescent • Human papillomavirus • Parental • Provider • Vaccination
- Vaccine hesitancy • Vaccine beliefs

KEY POINTS

- Misconceptions that contribute to parental vaccine hesitancy include that the human papillomavirus (HPV) vaccine is only relevant for girls/women, leads to promiscuity or sexual activity, and is unsafe.
- Safety concerns/side effects and lack of provider recommendation are the most common reasons for parental vaccine hesitancy.
- Health care providers, public health organizations, and others should address parental HPV vaccine hesitancy on many levels, incorporating discussion of vaccine misinformation currently circulating in the media (as needed by the specific parent) and addressing the historical context in racial/ethnic communities.
- Health care providers play a critical role in addressing HPV vaccine hesitancy because their recommendations influence hesitant parents.
- The presumptive recommendation approach has been found to be the most effective communication method to increase HPV vaccination uptake, but it may or may not address parental hesitancy in all cases.

INTRODUCTION

The first approved human papillomavirus (HPV) vaccine, a 4-valent vaccine targeting HPV types 6, 11, 16, and 18 (4vHPV), was licensed by the US Food and Drug Administration (FDA) in 2006 for use in females ages 9 through 26 years. The Advisory

[a] Department of Mexican American and Latino/a Studies, Latino Research Institute, The University of Texas at Austin, 210 West 24th Street, GWB 1.102, F9200, Austin, TX 78712, USA; [b] Department of Pediatrics, Indiana University School of Medicine, 410 West 10th Street, HS 1001, Indianapolis, IN 46202, USA; [c] Department of Pediatrics, Cincinnati Children's Hospital Medical Center, University of Cincinnati College of Medicine, 3333 Burnet Avenue, MLC 4000, Cincinnati, OH 45229, USA
* Corresponding author.
E-mail address: moralescampos@austin.utexas.edu

Pediatr Clin N Am 70 (2023) 211–226
https://doi.org/10.1016/j.pcl.2022.11.002   **pediatric.theclinics.com**
0031-3955/23/© 2022 Elsevier Inc. All rights reserved.

Committee on Immunization Practices (ACIP) issued a routine recommendation for female vaccination, with the targeted age range of 11 to 12 years to create a standardized platform for the tetanus, diphtheria, and pertussis (Tdap) booster; meningococcal ACWY; and HPV vaccines. In 2009 a 2-valent vaccine (2vHPV) targeting HPV types 16 and 18 was licensed for females and 4vHPV was licensed for males ages 9 through 26 years. In 2011 the ACIP recommended routine vaccination of males ages 9 through 21 years with 4vHPV. The vaccine was only routinely recommended for males ages 22 through 26 years who were immunocompromised or identified as men who have sex with men.[1] In 2014 a 9-valent vaccine was licensed by the FDA (9vHPV), replacing 4vHPV. Since 2016, 2vHPV has not been available in the United States. In 2019 the male and female age recommendations were harmonized so that routine vaccination was recommended for all individuals ages 9 through 26 years.[2] In 2022, the ACIP emphasized that routinely recommended HPV vaccination could begin at age 9 years.[3]

Currently, the only vaccine licensed and available in the United States is the 9-valent vaccine (9vHPV). Both 4vHPV and 9vHPV protect against HPV types 6 and 11, which are responsible for about 90% of genital warts. 9vHPV protects against 7 additional HPV types that have been causally associated with approximately 90% of cervical, anal, vaginal, vulvar, penile, and oropharyngeal cancers (types 16, 18, 31, 33, 45, 52, and 58).[4]

For this article, the authors define HPV vaccine hesitancy broadly as including attitudes or beliefs of doubt or concern about HPV vaccination, rather than only as HPV vaccine acceptance, delay, or rejection.[5] Hesitancy can lead to vaccination delay or refusal but can be present even when HPV vaccination is accepted at the recommended ages. Complete refusal to accept HPV vaccination, we would argue, is not an example of hesitancy, but reflects certainty, as misguided as it may be. Furthermore, a lack of hesitancy about HPV vaccination does not necessarily translate to HPV vaccine confidence. Many parents unhesitatingly accept HPV vaccination for their children/adolescents simply because a clinician has recommended it and these parents routinely follow the health care provider's recommendation regarding vaccination (**Fig. 1**). It is important to emphasize that assessment of hesitancy typically occurs at a single point in time and that persons all along the spectrum of HPV vaccine attitudes may change their stances with new information (or misinformation) or changing circumstances; this means that clinicians should not give up on confident rejectors and should not take confident acceptors for granted. Providers should check in with all parents regarding vaccination attitudes and need for information at every well-child and well-adolescent visit.

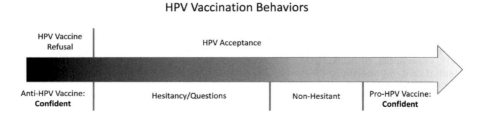

Fig. 1. HPV vaccination continuum.

HPV vaccine hesitancy is multifaceted. Individuals who are hesitant about all vaccines will certainly be hesitant about HPV vaccine. However, HPV vaccine hesitancy also has several unique features related to its history and to the fact that most HPV infections are sexually transmitted. There may be general hesitancy issues that take on salience with HPV vaccine (eg, questions about vaccine safety and/or effectiveness), but in this article the authors focus primarily on aspects of hesitancy that are unique to HPV vaccination.

They do not focus on the direct effect of policy approaches on vaccine coverage, such as school-entry requirements or school-located vaccination. These types of policies can have a profoundly positive impact on HPV vaccine uptake but are not designed to directly address hesitancy. At the same time, it is important to acknowledge that vaccination policy can indirectly affect hesitancy, and these potential indirect effects of policy are addressed here. This article largely addresses HPV vaccine hesitancy in the United States, although many of the issues that we identify may be relevant throughout North America and across other countries as well. Countries such as Canada, the United Kingdom, and Australia (among others) have approached HPV vaccination with very different implementation policies from those used by the United States. These HPV vaccination policy differences may have differential indirect effects on hesitancy.

The purpose of this review is to examine sources of HPV vaccine hesitancy among parents and providers to better understand and develop strategies to address them. In the following discussion the authors have organized their approach based on the 2014 report of the SAGE Working Group on Vaccine Hesitancy, which proposes 3 broad categories of determinants of hesitancy: contextual influences, individual and group influences, and vaccine/vaccination-specific issues.[6] Contextual influences include media, influential leaders, historical issues, and politics. Individual and group influences include beliefs, knowledge, social norms, and prior vaccination experiences. Vaccine/vaccination-specific issues include the strength and content of HPV vaccine recommendations by health care providers, the target of vaccination (ie, how the pathogen is transmitted; the lag time between infection and disease; and the severity of disease), and HPV vaccine policy (**Table 1**).

CONTEXTUAL INFLUENCES ON HUMAN PAPILLOMAVIRUS VACCINE HESITANCY

History of human papillomavirus vaccine hesitancy. Research on HPV vaccine acceptability just before and following licensure indicated high levels of acceptability, with approximately 80% of parents indicating that they would vaccinate their children, and with acceptance higher for older versus younger daughters and daughters versus sons.[7] Opposition to HPV vaccination was relatively muted, with even conservative religious groups not opposing vaccination but rejecting school-entry requirements. However, not long after the FDA-licensed 4vHPV and the ACIP recommended it in 2006, several states began to consider legislation that would require HPV vaccination for girls entering middle school.[8–10] These efforts, which were highlighted by Texas governor Rick Perry's executive order in 2007 to require HPV vaccination (an order that was overruled by the state legislature), generated a great deal of controversy. The controversy grew more intense when it was revealed that the manufacturer of 4vHPV was involved in working with state legislators to pass school-entry requirements. Ultimately, these issues led to a backlash against HPV vaccination and may have significantly increased hesitancy around the vaccine, due in part to the negative media coverage that ensued.

Table 1
Adapted World Health Organization working group determinants of human papillomavirus vaccine hesitancy

Contextual Influences Influences arising due to historical, sociocultural, environmental, or political factors	• Communication and media environment • Influential leaders, immunization program gatekeepers and anti-or pro-vaccination lobbies. • Historical influences • Religion/culture/gender/socio-economic • Politics/policies • Perception of the pharmaceutical industry
Individual and Group Influences Influences arising from personal perception of the vaccine or influences of the social/peer environment	• Personal, family, and/or community members' experience with vaccination, including pain • Beliefs, attitudes about health and prevention • Beliefs related to a child's sexual behavior • Knowledge/awareness • Health system and provider's trust and personal experience • Risk/benefit (perceived, heuristic)
Vaccine/Vaccination-Specific Issues Directly related to vaccine or vaccination	• Effectiveness of the vaccine • Concerns about vaccine safety • Risk/Benefit (epidemiologic and scientific evidence) • The strength of the recommendation and/or knowledge base and/or attitude of health care professionals

Another unique set of issues particularly relevant to HPV vaccination were the frequent changes in licensure indications and recommendations over the years since the vaccine was first approved in the United States in 2006 (**Table 2**). HPV vaccination was first approved and routinely recommended for females only. After multiple changes in guidance over the intervening years, the recommendations for females and males were not fully harmonized until 2019, 13 years after initial approval. The frequent changes in licensure and recommendations, although driven by emerging research, may have confused primary care clinicians, resulting in decreased confidence (increased hesitancy) in recommending HPV vaccination. The delay in harmonizing the recommendations for men and females also created confusion about the nature of HPV infection, disease, and vaccination, with many parents believing HPV to be mainly a female issue (ie, what has been called the feminization of HPV).[11] As a result, some parents, to this day, do not realize that HPV vaccination has direct benefit for their sons.[12]

Communication and media environment. Many research articles have focused on the ways in which information about HPV vaccines is presented on social media sites and the influence of social media on attitudes about HPV vaccination.[13] Studies[12,14–17] of the association between media and HPV vaccine hesitancy indicate that parents rely on the media for information but also recognize it may contain misinformation and note that messaging must be tailored to address specific concerns. Using national immunization data (2015–2018), Sonawane and colleagues[18] showed an increase in

Table 2
History of human papillomavirus vaccine policies

Year	Authorization	Recommendations for Females	Recommendations for Males
2006	Three-dose series of *4vHPV* indicated for females ages 9–26 y for prevention of cervical, vulvar, and vaginal cancers and genital warts	Three-dose series of *4vHPV* routinely recommended for females ages 11–12 y. Routine catch-up recommendation for females ages 13–26 y. "Permissive" recommendation for females ages 9–10 y	
2009	Three-dose series of *2vHPV* indicated for females ages 9–26 y for prevention of cervical cancers and precancers	Three-dose series of *2vHPV* routinely recommended for females ages 11–12 y. Routine catch-up recommendation for females ages 13–26 y. "Permissive" recommendation for females ages 9–10 y	
2009	Three-dose series of *4vHPV* indicated for males ages 9–26 y for prevention of genital warts	Unchanged	"Permissive" recommendation of three-dose series of *4vHPV* for males
2011	Three-dose series of *4vHPV* indicated for females and males ages 9–26 y for prevention of anal cancers and precancers	Unchanged	Three-dose series of *4vHPV* routinely recommended for males ages 11–12 y. Routine catch-up vaccination for males ages 13–21 y. Permissive recommendation for males ages 9–10 and 22–26 y. Routine recommendation for males ages 22–26 y who are immunocompromised or are men who have sex with men (MSM)
2014	Three-dose series of *9vHPV* indicated for females and males ages 9–26 y for prevention of cervical, vulvar, vaginal, and anal cancers and genital warts. Gradually replaces *4vHPV*	Unchanged	Unchanged

(continued on next page)

Table 2
(continued)

Year	Authorization	Recommendations for Females	Recommendations for Males
2016	—	Two-dose series of 9vHPV and 2vHPV recommended if the first dose is given before age 15 y. When the first dose is given at age 15 y or older, the three-dose is still recommended	Two-dose series of 9vHPV recommended if the first dose is given before age 15 y. When the first dose is given at ages 15–21 y, the three-dose is still recommended for routine catch-up vaccination. Routine recommendation only for males ages 22–26 y who are immunocompromised, are MSM, or are transgender persons
2016	2vHPV withdrawn from the US market by the manufacturer	—	—
2019	—	Unchanged	Recommendations of 9vHPV for males through age 26 y harmonized with recommendations for females
2019	9vHPV indicated for use in persons ages 27–45 y	Shared clinical decision-making recommendation of 9vHPV for ages 27–45 y	Shared clinical decision-making recommendation of 9vHPV for ages 27–45 y
2020	9vHPV indicated for prevention of HPV-related oropharyngeal and other head and neck cancers	Unchanged	Unchanged
2021	—	Can begin routine recommendation of 9vHPV at ages 9–10 y	Can begin routine recommendation of 9vHPV at ages 9–10 y

the proportion of parents who refused the HPV vaccine for their adolescents due to safety concerns over time. They noted this may have resulted from unsubstantiated HPV vaccine–related adverse event reports on social media and online blogs. Walker and colleagues[12] (2020) interviewed 30 mothers in the Mid-West and found that respondents viewed the media as the main source of HPV vaccination confusion, misinformation, and fear. Interestingly, these same mothers believed the media should address these fears by providing accurate statistics on safety and adverse side effects and information about vaccine benefits, such as protection against cancer. Similarly, Latina mothers in a study conducted by Lindsay and colleagues[19] suggested several strategies to promote uptake of the HPV vaccine, which included social media distribution of personal narratives that reduce parents' HPV vaccination hesitancy. Of note, findings from Argyris and colleagues'[20] analysis of antivaccine versus provaccine social media posts indicated that antivaccine posts were associated with increased vaccine hesitancy and decreases in their children's HPV vaccination rates, whereas provaccine content had no association with either.

There have been recent efforts[21–23] to develop strategies to counter online/social media misinformation about HPV vaccination, including training HPV vaccine–confident parents to post supportive comments on their social media accounts. However, much more needs to be done, and other stakeholders, in addition to parents, need to be strategically active on social media, to help neutralize the negative impact of misinformation.[24,25] These stakeholders include primary care practices and health systems (Please see the article by Hoffman and colleagues "Social Media and Vaccine Hesitancy: Help Us Move the Needle" in this issue of the journal.)

Religious factors. According to the Pew Research Center,[26,27] almost 77% of US adults affiliate with a religious faith and 53% state that religion is important to them. Public health efforts aimed at improving vaccination rates need to consider beliefs of different faith groups and tailor interventions appropriately. Religious communities and leaders have often been hesitant to mandate or strongly recommend the vaccine because HPV is sexually transmitted and there is the perception that actively supporting vaccination will be interpreted as condoning premarital sexual activity.[27] However, research shows clearly there is no evidence of increased sexual risk outcomes following HPV vaccination among adolescents.[28,29]

INDIVIDUAL AND GROUP INFLUENCES

Personal, family, and/or community members' experience with vaccination. The social norms and values present within a culture, in addition to the lived experience of an individual and those persons within their close social network, may also affect HPV vaccine hesitancy.[30] Callaghan and colleagues[31] found in their parent survey investigating predictors of delayed vaccination that needle sensitivity was significantly associated with delayed HPV vaccination. Parents who experience high anxiety and discomfort with needles, in extreme cases leading to panic or fainting, may be more likely to experience the same anxiety when having to vaccinate their child. Sundstrom and colleagues[23] also reported that hesitant parents described hearing comments about injuries and deaths related to the HPV vaccine and that these comments influenced their decision to delay.

Parental beliefs and attitudes about health and prevention. Szilagyi and colleagues[32] found in their sample of US parents that some did not believe the HPV vaccine was beneficial for their child, protected against HPV-related cancer, or was effective. In all, 23% of the sample were deemed to be hesitant about HPV vaccination, based on their scores on an HPV Vaccine Hesitancy Scale. Pomares and colleagues[33] studied individuals' general cognitive biases (ie, not specific to vaccination), including base rate neglect, conjunction fallacy, sunk cost fallacy, present bias, risk aversion, and information avoidance. They reported that 2 of the cognitive biases may be positively associated with greater parental vaccine hesitancy:

- *Information avoidance* (preference to not to obtain knowledge that is freely available, especially if that knowledge is unwanted or unpleasant, for example, could threaten one's ideas or beliefs)
- *Present bias* (tendency to give stronger weight to more-immediate payoffs than long-term payoffs)

In contrast, their findings indicated an association with *lower* vaccine hesitancy in the presence of individuals prone to 2 other cognitive biases:

- *Conjunction fallacy* (when an individual perceives a specific condition as more likely than a general condition, of which it is a subset)
- *Sunk cost bias* (individuals are compelled to continue a behavior toward a goal, for example, continuing to vaccinate according to the recommended schedule, because they have previously invested resources)

Anther cognitive bias, omission bias, has been studied with vaccination in general and may apply, as well, to HPV vaccination.[34] Omission bias refers to the tendency to attribute more sense of responsibility for negative outcomes to acts of commission (eg, concern about side effects due to getting one's child vaccinated) than to acts of omission (eg, concern about infection or disease due to not getting one's child vaccinated).[34]

Francis and colleagues[35] surveyed providers to learn more about their experience with vaccine-hesitant parents and providers' confidence in responding to their concerns. The results of the study showed that providers were least confident in responding to parents' religious or personal beliefs.

Knowledge and awareness about human papillomavirus and human papillomavirus vaccines. One of the most common reasons for parental HPV vaccine refusal is lack of knowledge regarding the HPV vaccine or awareness of HPV. Lack of knowledge/awareness about the vaccine and the disease may leave parents susceptible to misinformation and misconceptions about vaccines.[30] Thompson and colleagues[36] examined National Immunization Survey-Teen 2012 to 2015 data and found that parental lack of knowledge was significantly more likely to be the reason for nonvaccination in 2012 to 2013, and parents were significantly less likely to use this reason for female compared with male children; this may be related to the feminization of HPV and late recommendation of the vaccine for men. Khodadadi and colleagues[37] found that among Latina mothers higher HPV vaccine awareness was associated with greater willingness to accept vaccination. The study also demonstrated that parents who have more education are more likely to refuse[38] or delay[39] HPV vaccination than those with less education. Parents with less education may rely on the practitioner to evaluate the risks and benefits of the vaccine.

Providers addressing parental lack of knowledge through follow-up counseling is important because secondary acceptance (vaccinating after initially refusing or delaying) is common.[40] In a study by Kornides and colleagues,[40] the investigators analyzed data from a national survey of parents who declined HPV vaccination but accepted the vaccine at a subsequent visit. The parents reported one of their reasons for acceptance was that they learned more about the vaccine through counseling by their provider. According to Patel and colleagues,[41] the knowledge and attitudes of health care providers toward vaccination are reflected in parental attitudes toward vaccinations; thus, positive engagement between providers and parents is essential. A review by Bratic and colleagues[42] also showed that HPV vaccine knowledge and acceptance are inconsistent among providers, so better professional training may be needed.

Beliefs related to a child's sexual behavior. Research on HPV vaccine hesitancy suggests that parents' beliefs regarding sexual purity and chastity before marriage—both of which may be related to their religious beliefs—are key to their decisions regarding HPV vaccination. Beliefs related to a child's sexual behavior are important to consider when addressing parents' decisions to refuse or delay vaccination.[31,38,43] For example, Callaghan and colleagues[31] define "moral purity" as a belief that leads "persons to avoid perceived bodily contamination and individuals, objects, and experiences that violate sanctity or self-control." The investigators demonstrated that parents who highly valued "moral purity" were more likely to delay vaccination compared with those who had lower scores. Parents with higher scores were more likely to hold conservative beliefs about sexuality, thus were less likely to believe vaccinating children/preadolescents against HPV was proper[31] or necessary before sexual activity.[38] According to Bratic and colleagues,[42] hesitancy may stem from parental concerns that the physician's recommendation may lead to discussion with their child about sexual activity in the office. As noted earlier, other parents may be concerned that their vaccinated adolescent would be more inclined to initiate sexual activity but there is no evidence of increased sexual activity among vaccinated adolescents.[28,29] Butterfield and colleagues[38] also noted that parents who had a history of sexually transmitted infections were more likely to agree to vaccinate. In Francis and colleagues'[35] survey, providers were asked about their level of confidence responding to parents in various settings. More providers (64%) reported feeling very confident in discussing the appropriateness of recommending the HPV vaccine for a child who is *not* sexually active than in other scenarios, for example, the parent has concerns about the vaccine's safety or side effects; it is not mandatory for school. This provider confidence is critical in alleviating parental concerns about a child being too young for HPV vaccine.

Trust in the health system and providers. (Please see the article on culture in this issue of the journal.) Many racial/ethnic groups (eg, African American, Hispanic, Native American) have a history of medical distrust and trauma stemming from negative experiences with the US government and other institutions as well as researchers and physicians. These negative experiences included the Tuskegee study, involuntary sterilization of Latinas in California and Puerto Rico and of Native women, and discriminatory health policies, which may contribute to HPV vaccine hesitancy among these groups.[44–46] Tsui and colleagues,[45] for example, reported that in a study of largely Hispanic/Latino parents, there was an association between high levels of medical mistrust and HPV vaccine hesitancy. In a study conducted by Szilagyi and colleagues,[32] a high proportion of mixed-race parents reported distrusting the HPV vaccine information they received from their adolescent's health care provider.

Perceived risks and benefits of vaccination. In Khodadadi and colleagues'[37] study of Latina mothers, greater HPV vaccine hesitancy was associated with lower perceived self-risk of cervical cancer, lower HPV awareness, lower perceived risk of HPV among daughters, lower perceived self-efficacy score to complete the vaccination series, and having health insurance for their daughter. In a study of providers, Cunningham-Erves and collegaues[39] reported that some of the most common reasons for parental vaccine hesitancy as perceived by providers were the child being too young and at low risk of HPV infection through sexual activity.

VACCINE/VACCINATION-SPECIFIC ISSUES

Concerns about vaccine safety and infertility. Despite numerous studies demonstrating that HPV vaccines are safe and well tolerated, many parents are concerned about HPV vaccine safety, especially long-term side effects that may not become apparent until later in life.[23,32,39,47,48] Thomas and colleagues[49] demonstrated that in a survey of parents in rural south Florida, 80% believed HPV vaccination could leave their child sterile. Studies also have revealed gender differences regarding concerns about safety and side effects. Thompson and colleagues[36] reported that parents of females were more likely to state they were concerned about safety and side effects compared with those of males (odds ratio [OR] = 2.19, 95% confidence interval [CI], 1.98–2.41). Parents tend to turn to their providers with their safety concerns[50] (eg, the vaccine causing infertility or sudden death), but Francis and colleagues[35] reported (when looking at individual items) that providers in their study were less confident responding to parents' concerns regarding lasting than acute health problems thought to be caused by the HPV vaccine.

Risk/Benefit Assessment. Bratic and colleagues[42] reported that parents may prioritize the HPV vaccine lower than other childhood vaccines because it offers delayed benefits and no perceived short-term benefit for their children. Patel and colleagues[41] found in their review of parental hesitancy that parents were more concerned with potential morbidity and mortality of HPV-associated diseases, rather than the sexually transmitted nature of the HPV infection.

INCREASING HUMAN PAPILLOMAVIRUS VACCINE ACCEPTANCE AND UPTAKE

When parents express vaccine hesitancy, regardless of the reason, it is critical for providers to focus on respectful dialogue, strongly recommend the HPV vaccine, and respond to specific questions or concerns.[51] Butterfield and colleagues[38] reported that the following factors correlate with an increased rate of vaccine acceptance: strong HPV vaccine recommendation from a provider; recommendation of concurrently required adolescent vaccines at the same time as the HPV vaccine; discussion of the benefits of vaccination; and discussion of these issues using a positive tone. Shay and colleagues[51] reported that parental vaccine hesitancy was subject to positive influence and that undecided parents, who made assertive statements about their vaccine hesitancy, were still amenable to vaccination when providers responded to hesitancy by endorsing the vaccine with a brief rationale.

Gilkey and colleagues[52] conducted a study measuring the quality of provider recommendation using 3 indicators with a value of one point each: stating it is important to receive, highlighting that it prevents HPV-related cancers, and stressing the urgency of same day vaccination. The investigators found that high-quality recommendations (2 to 3 points) were associated with an increase in vaccination initiation. In a study by Lockhart and colleagues,[53] medical staff reported that learning a presumptive approach (ie, assuming the parent intends to vaccinate) and motivational interviewing skills benefited them in communicating with HPV vaccine–hesitant parent because they were better equipped for these types of challenging conversations. Similarly, medical providers in a mixed methods study by Newcomer and colleagues[50] identified the following as facilitators of HPV vaccination: using a presumptive style of recommending the vaccine, offering the HPV vaccine with recommended vaccines, and emphasizing the HPV vaccine as a tool for cancer prevention. Dempsey and colleagues[54] conducted a study of parental report of provider HPV communication strategies used as part of a randomized control trial. The investigators found that receipt of a presumptive recommendation was associated with a lower likelihood of having concerns about the vaccine's safety, lower vaccine hesitancy, and an increased likelihood of vaccination. Several studies have also found that training clinicians in communication strategies can improve vaccination rates but also reduce missed opportunities.[55–58] As noted by Opel article in this journal, there are communication strategies clinicians can use for HPV vaccine hesitancy that are important to be aware of and can include motivational interviewing. Following is a table of resources and scripts for clinicians (**Box 1**).

DISCUSSION

This review examined available evidence on HPV vaccine hesitancy among parents and providers, framing results in 3 categories: contextual, individual and group, and vaccine/vaccination-specific issues. The most consistently identified determinants of HPV vaccine hesitancy in the literature include media misinformation, lack of knowledge and awareness about HPV and HPV vaccines, belief that HPV vaccines are not necessary before initiating sexual activity, concerns about adolescents initiating or increasing sexual activity postvaccination (ie, risk compensation), parental concerns about vaccine effectiveness and safety, and lack of strong provider recommendation. Evidence-based strategies to address these determinants include education of parents about HPV and HPV vaccines; education of providers about reliable health resources for parents, ACIP guidelines, and vaccine efficacy; and ensuring that providers offer strong vaccine recommendations at every contact with adolescent patients. Providers' use of a presumptive recommendation approach for HPV vaccination increases uptake of vaccine but may or may not address hesitancy. Strategies to address vaccine hesitancy should consider not only vaccine misinformation but also the broader historical contexts that can result in parental mistrust in providers and health care systems. Of course, lack of access to preventative services in medically underserved areas must be addressed. Coupling high-quality provider recommendations and communication strategies with practice changes has the potential to decrease hesitancy and increase confidence in HPV vaccination, and this may increase HPV vaccination rates so that

---

Box 1
Clinician resources for communication trainings and example videos with scripts

Free application for iPhones and Android phones called "HPV vaccine: Same Way, Same Day" that provides interactive training in MI techniques
- Android: https://play.google.com/store/apps/details?id=com.kognito.hpv_immunization_update
- Apple: https://apps.apple.com/us/app/hpv-vaccine-same-way-same-day/id1356847181

Maintenance of Certification (MOC) training on HPV vaccination available through the Indiana Immunization Coalition that is approved by the American Board of Pediatrics and the American Board of Family Medicine and available to physicians across the United States. https://vaccinateindiana.org/hpv-moc/

UNITY United for adolescent vaccination has resources for Healthcare Providers https://www.unity4teenvax.org/health-care-providers/

National HPV Vaccination Roundtable Resource for Clinicians. https://hpvroundtable.org/resource-library/#filter=.clinicians

Centers for Disease Control and Prevention has clinician video series on effective strategies on recommending HPV vaccination to parents of adolescents. https://www.cdc.gov/vaccines/howirecommend/adolescent-vacc-videos.html

we reach the Healthy People 2030 goal and decrease hesitancy and increase confidence in HPV vaccination.

Further research that could guide the development of effective interventions to reduce HPV vaccine hesitancy are as follows:

- Future studies on laws or mandates and recommendation guidelines in different states could provide lessons on how policy drives provider practice and patient actions and influences hesitancy.
- Further examination of the roles of culture, historical context/trauma, and social networks of specific communities would better inform us on how interventions can be designed to decrease vaccine hesitancy.
- Developing and testing interventions to counter online/social media misinformation about HPV vaccination has high potential to reduce vaccine hesitancy.
- Training health care providers to be vaccine advocates and equipping them with facts and scripts to help respond to parent/patient questions and concerns may help to alleviate parental anxiety about the HPV vaccine.
- Further research should address which multistrategy and multilevel interventions are most effective in sustaining increased rates for HPV vaccination and boosting confidence.[48]

CLINICS CARE POINTS

- Pediatricians and other primary care providers should be aware that most parents will accept HPV vaccination for their children and adolescents but that acceptance does not preclude ongoing hesitancy about HPV vaccination.
- For children ages 9 and 10 years and younger adolescents, parents should be the primary (although not sole) focus of HPV vaccination discussions. However, for older adolescents, it is important for clinicians to recognize that these adolescents may have an increased role in HPV vaccine decision-making and may hold unique beliefs, different from their parents, related to vaccine hesitancy and confidence.
- Through anticipatory guidance and vaccine recommendations, primary care providers play a critical role in increasing confidence in—and reducing hesitancy about—HPV vaccination.
- Parents encounter a great deal of misinformation about HPV vaccination on social media sites, and primary care providers should be prepared to ask parents about sources of information and to answer parental questions/concerns about HPV vaccine in a nonjudgmental manner.
- Pediatricians and other primary care providers should be cognizant of their own hesitancy about recommending HPV vaccination and take steps to reduce hesitancy (and increase confidence) in their communications to parents and patients.

DISCLOSURES

D.Y. Morales-Campos and J.A. Kahn have no conflicts of interest. G.D. Zimet reports serving as an advisory board member for Pfizer and Moderna and as a consultant for Merck, United States. He also receives research funding from Merck administered through Indiana University, United States.

REFERENCES

1. Centers for Disease Control and Prevention. Recommendations on the use of quadrivalent human papillomavirus vaccine in males–Advisory Committee on Immunization Practices (ACIP). MMWR Morb Mortal Wkly Rep 2011;60(50):1705–8.

2. Meites E, Szilagyi PG, Chesson HW, et al. Human papillomavirus vaccination for adults: updated recommendations of the advisory committee on immunization practices. MMWR Morb Mortal Wkly Rep 2019;68:698–702.
3. Centers for Disease and Control and Prevention. Child and adolescent immunization schedule, recommendations for ages 18 years of younger, United States. 2022. Available at: https://www.cdc.gov/vaccines/schedules/hcp/imz/child-adolescent.html. Accessed July 29, 2022.
4. Senkomago V, Henley SJ, Thomas CC, et al. Human papillomavirus-attributable cancers - United States, 2012-2016. MMWR Morb Mortal Wkly Rep 2019; 68(33):724–8.
5. Larson HJ, Gakidou E, Murray CJL. The vaccine-hesitant moment. N Engl J Med 2022;387(1):58–65.
6. Strategic advisory group of experts (SAGE) Working Group on Vaccine Hesitancy Report of the SAGE Working Group on Vaccine Hesitancy. 2014. Available at: https://www.asset-scienceinsociety.eu/sites/default/files/sage_working_group_revised_report_vaccine_hesitancy.pdf. Accessed July 28, 2022.
7. Kahn JA, Ding L, Huang B, et al. Mothers' intention for their daughters and themselves to receive the human papillomavirus vaccine: a national study of nurses. Pediatrics 2009;123(6):1439–45.
8. Udesky L. Push to mandate HPV vaccine triggers backlash in USA. Lancet 2007; 369(9566):979–80.
9. Haber G, Malow RM, Zimet GD. The HPV vaccine mandate controversy. J Pediatr Adolesc Gynecol 2007;20(6):325–31.
10. Colgrove J, Abiola S, Mello MM. HPV vaccination mandates–lawmaking amid political and scientific controversy. N Engl J Med 2010;363(8):785–91.
11. Daley EM, Vamos CA, Zimet GD, et al. The feminization of HPV: reversing gender biases in us human papillomavirus vaccine policy. Am J Public Health 2016; 106(6):983–4.
12. Walker KK, Owens H, Zimet G. "We fear the unknown": emergence, route and transfer of hesitancy and misinformation among HPV vaccine accepting mothers. Prev Med Rep 2020;20:101240.
13. Ortiz RR, Smith A, Coyne-Beasley T. A systematic literature review to examine the potential for social media to impact HPV vaccine uptake and awareness, knowledge, and attitudes about HPV and HPV vaccination. Hum Vaccin Immunother 2019;15(7–8):1465–75.
14. Walker KK, Owens H, Zimet G. The role of the media on maternal confidence in provider HPV recommendation. BMC Public Health 2020;20(1):1765.
15. Zhang J, Xue H, Calabrese C, et al. Understanding human papillomavirus vaccine promotions and hesitancy in northern california through examining public facebook pages and groups. Front Digit Health 2021;3:683090.
16. Dilley SE, Peral S, Straughn JM Jr, et al. The challenge of HPV vaccination uptake and opportunities for solutions: lessons learned from Alabama. Prev Med 2018; 113:124–31.
17. Painter JE, Viana De OMS, Jimenez L, et al. Vaccine-related attitudes and decision-making among uninsured, Latin American immigrant mothers of adolescent daughters: a qualitative study. Hum Vaccin Immunother 2019;15(1):121–33.
18. Sonawane K, Lin YY, Damgacioglu H, et al. Trends in human papillomavirus vaccine safety concerns and adverse event reporting in the United States. JAMA Netw Open 2021;4(9):e2124502.
19. Lindsay AC, Delgado D, Valdez MJ, et al. "Everyone in our community should be informed about the human papillomavirus vaccine": Latinx Mothers' Suggested

Strategies to Promote the Human Papillomavirus Vaccine. Am J Health Promot 2022;36(5):853–63.

20. Argyris YA, Kim Y, Roscizewski A, et al. The mediating role of vaccine hesitancy between maternal engagement with anti- and pro-vaccine social media posts and adolescent HPV-vaccine uptake rates in the US: The perspective of loss aversion in emotion-laden decision circumstances. Soc Sci Med 2021;282: 114043.

21. Buller DB, Pagoto S, Henry K, et al. Human papillomavirus vaccination and social media: results in a trial with mothers of daughters aged 14-17. Front Digit Health 2021;3:683034.

22. Sundstrom B, Cartmell KB, White AA, et al. Correcting HPV vaccination misinformation online: evaluating the. Vaccines (Basel) 2021;9(4). https://doi.org/10.3390/vaccines9040352.

23. Sundstrom B, Cartmell KB, White AA, et al. HPV vaccination champions: evaluating a technology-mediated intervention for parents. Front Digit Health 2021;3: 636161.

24. Hoffman BL, Felter EM, Chu KH, et al. It's not all about autism: the emerging landscape of anti-vaccination sentiment on Facebook. Vaccine 2019;37(16):2216–23.

25. Steffens MS, Dunn AG, Leask J, et al. Using social media for vaccination promotion: practices and challenges. Digit Health 2020;6. 2055207620970785.

26. Pew Research Center. U.S. Public becoming less religious. 2015. Available at: https://www.pewresearch.org/religion/2015/11/03/u-s-public-becoming-less-religious/. Accessed July 22, 2022.

27. Muravsky NL, Betesh GM, McCoy RG. Religious doctrine and attitudes toward vaccination in Jewish Law. J Relig Health 2021;1–16. https://doi.org/10.1007/s10943-021-01447-8.

28. Madhivanan P, Pierre-Victor D, Mukherjee S, et al. Human papillomavirus vaccination and sexual disinhibition in females: a systematic review. Am J Prev Med 2016;51(3):373–83.

29. Zimet GD, Rosberger Z, Fisher WA, et al. Beliefs, behaviors and HPV vaccine: correcting the myths and the misinformation. Prev Med 2013;57(5):414–8.

30. Maisonneuve AR, Witteman HO, Brehaut J, et al. Educating children and adolescents about vaccines: a review of current literature. Expert Rev Vaccines 2018; 17(4):311–21.

31. Callaghan T, Motta M, Sylvester S, et al. Parent psychology and the decision to delay childhood vaccination. Soc Sci Med 2019;238:112407.

32. Szilagyi PG, Albertin CS, Gurfinkel D, et al. Prevalence and characteristics of HPV vaccine hesitancy among parents of adolescents across the US. Vaccine 2020; 38(38):6027–37.

33. Pomares TD, Buttenheim AM, Amin AB, et al. Association of cognitive biases with human papillomavirus vaccine hesitancy: a cross-sectional study. Hum Vaccin Immunother 2020;16(5):1018–23.

34. Sherman GD, Vallen B, Finkelstein SR, et al. When taking action means accepting responsibility: omission bias predicts parents' reluctance to vaccinate due to greater anticipated culpability for negative side effects. J Consum Aff 2021; 55(4):1660–81.

35. Francis JKR, Rodriguez SA, Dorsey O, et al. Provider perspectives on communication and dismissal policies with HPV vaccine hesitant parents. Prev Med Rep 2021;24:101562.

36. Thompson EL, Rosen BL, Vamos CA, et al. Human papillomavirus vaccination: what are the reasons for nonvaccination among U.S. Adolescents? J Adolesc Health 2017;61(3):288–93.
37. Khodadadi AB, Redden DT, Scarinci IC. HPV vaccination hesitancy among latina immigrant mothers despite physician recommendation. Ethn Dis Fall 2020;30(4): 661–70.
38. Butterfield R, Dhanani S. The development of human papillomavirus (HPV) vaccines and current barriers to implementation. Immunol Invest 2021;50(7):821–32.
39. Cunningham-Erves J, Koyama T, Huang Y, et al. Providers' perceptions of parental human papillomavirus vaccine hesitancy: cross-sectional study. JMIR Cancer 2019;5(2):e13832.
40. Kornides ML, McRee AL, Gilkey MB. Parents who decline HPV vaccination: who later accepts and why? Acad Pediatr 2018;18(2s):S37–43.
41. Patel PR, Berenson AB. Sources of HPV vaccine hesitancy in parents. Hum Vaccin Immunother 2013;9(12):2649–53.
42. Bratic JS, Seyferth ER, Bocchini JA Jr. Update on barriers to human papillomavirus vaccination and effective strategies to promote vaccine acceptance. Curr Opin Pediatr 2016;28(3):407–12.
43. Yankey D, Elam-Evans LD, Bish CL, et al. Human papillomavirus vaccination estimates among adolescents in the mississippi delta region: national immunization survey-teen, 2015-2017. Prev Chronic Dis 2020;17:E31.
44. Bordeaux SJ, Baca AW, Begay RL, et al. Designing Inclusive HPV cancer vaccines and increasing uptake among native americans-a cultural perspective review. Curr Oncol 2021;28(5):3705–16.
45. Tsui J, Martinez B, Shin MB, et al. Understanding medical mistrust and HPV vaccine hesitancy among multiethnic parents in Los Angeles. J Behav Med 2022;1–16. https://doi.org/10.1007/s10865-022-00283-9.
46. Stern AM. Sterilized in the name of public health: race, immigration, and reproductive control in modern California. Am J Public Health 2005;95(7):1128–38.
47. Gualano MR, Olivero E, Voglino G, et al. Knowledge, attitudes and beliefs towards compulsory vaccination: a systematic review. Hum Vaccin Immunother 2019;15(4):918–31.
48. Holloway GL. Effective HPV vaccination strategies: what does the evidence say? an integrated literature review. J Pediatr Nurs 2019;44:31–41.
49. Thomas TL, Caldera M, Maurer J. A short report: parents HPV vaccine knowledge in rural South Florida. Hum Vaccin Immunother 2019;15(7–8):1666–71.
50. Newcomer SR, Caringi J, Jones B, et al. A mixed-methods analysis of barriers to and facilitators of human papillomavirus vaccination among adolescents in Montana. Public Health Rep 2020;135(6):842–50.
51. Shay LA, Baldwin AS, Betts AC, et al. Parent-provider communication of HPV vaccine hesitancy. Pediatrics 2018;141(6). https://doi.org/10.1542/peds.2017-2312.
52. Gilkey MB, Calo WA, Marciniak MW, et al. Parents who refuse or delay HPV vaccine: differences in vaccination behavior, beliefs, and clinical communication preferences. Hum Vaccin Immunother 2017;13(3):680–6.
53. Lockhart S, Dempsey AF, Pyrzanowski J, et al. Provider and parent perspectives on enhanced communication tools for human papillomavirus vaccine-hesitant parents. Acad Pediatr 2018;18(7):776–82.
54. Dempsey AF, Pyrzanowski J, Campagna EJ, et al. Parent report of provider HPV vaccine communication strategies used during a randomized, controlled trial of a provider communication intervention. Vaccin 2019;37(10):1307–12.

55. Dempsey AF, Pyrznawoski J, Lockhart S, et al. Effect of a health care professional communication training intervention on adolescent human papillomavirus vaccination: a cluster randomized clinical trial. JAMA Pediatr 2018;172(5):e180016.
56. Szilagyi PG, Humiston SG, Stephens-Shields AJ, et al. Effect of training pediatric clinicians in human papillomavirus communication strategies on human papillomavirus vaccination rates: a cluster randomized clinical trial. JAMA Pediatr 2021;175(9):901–10.
57. Limaye RJ, Opel DJ, Dempsey A, et al. Communicating with vaccine-hesitant parents: a narrative review. Acad Pediatr 2021;21(4S):S24–9.
58. Rand CM, Humiston SG. Provider focused interventions to improve child and adolescent vaccination rates. Acad Pediatr 2021;21(4S):S34–9.

Influenza Vaccine Hesitancy
Scope, Influencing Factors, and Strategic Interventions

Ashley B. Stephens, MD[a], Annika M. Hofstetter, MD, PhD, MPH[b,c],
Melissa S. Stockwell, MD, MPH[a,d],*

KEYWORDS

- Influenza • Influenza vaccine • Vaccine hesitancy • Interventions • Informatics

KEY POINTS

- We discuss current influenza vaccination coverage for children, which is suboptimal and decreased during the last season.
- We describe influenza vaccine hesitancy and tools to effectively measure it.
- We introduce the adapted "Intent to Vaccinate Model" as a framework to understand and address influenza vaccine hesitancy.
- We discuss several interventions that address "what people think and feel," "social processes," and "practical issues" that can help increase influenza vaccine uptake.

INTRODUCTION

Vaccine hesitancy is not a new phenomenon. It has existed since just after the creation of the first vaccine against smallpox by Edward Jenner in England in the late 1700s.[1,2] Vaccine hesitancy exists on a spectrum not only for the level of hesitancy but also across different vaccines. Influenza vaccine often stands alone in the vaccine hesitancy realm, with many people who have little hesitancy in getting other vaccines choosing not be vaccinated against influenza.[3]

Influenza vaccine was developed in the 1940s, initially as a vaccine to protect against influenza A and later as a vaccine to protect against influenza A and B.[4] At first, influenza vaccine was only available to those enlisted in the military but it was soon

[a] Division of Child and Adolescent Health, Department of Pediatrics, Columbia University, Vagelos College of Physicians and Surgeons and NewYork-Presbyterian, 622 West 168th Street - VC 417, New York, NY 10032, USA; [b] Department of Pediatrics, University of Washington School of Medicine, 1959 NE Pacific Street, Seattle, WA 981952, USA; [c] Seattle Children's Research Institute, M/S CURE-4, PO Box 5371, Seattle, WA 98145, USA; [d] Department of Population and Family Health, Mailman School of Public Health, Columbia University, 60 Haven Avenue, New York, NY 10032, USA
* Corresponding author. 622 West 168th Street - VC 417, New York, NY 10032.
E-mail address: mss2112@cumc.columbia.edu

Pediatr Clin N Am 70 (2023) 227–241
https://doi.org/10.1016/j.pcl.2022.11.003
0031-3955/23/© 2022 Elsevier Inc. All rights reserved.
pediatric.theclinics.com

after licensed for civilian adults.[4] It was recommended for children aged 6 through 23 months in 2002, for children aged 24 to 59 months in 2006, and for children aged 5 to 18 years in 2008.[4] There are particular characteristics of influenza vaccine that make it more prone to hesitancy, including the fact that influenza vaccine effectiveness against symptomatic disease is lower than that of other vaccines, the vaccine is required annually, and there are specific false beliefs related to the influenza vaccine.[5] In this commentary, we aim to discuss influenza vaccine hesitancy, including tools to assess for it, factors that influence it, and interventions that could be used to improve influenza vaccine uptake.

Influenza Vaccination Coverage

Influenza vaccination is important in preventing hospitalizations and deaths in children. For high-severity seasons, such as the 2017 to 18 influenza season, influenza vaccination was estimated to have averted more than 2.1 million illnesses, 1.4 million medical visits, 14,790 hospitalizations, and 41 deaths to 74 deaths among young children (aged 6 months to 4 years) and more than 1.3 million illnesses, 710,000 medical visits, 3,700 hospitalizations, and 15 deaths to 89 deaths among children aged 5 to 17 years.[6] The Advisory Committee on Immunization Practices recommends that all children aged 6 months and older without contraindications receive annual influenza vaccine; some children who are 6 months through 8 years need 2 doses in a given season, depending on their previous vaccination status.[7]

Rates of annual influenza vaccination coverage of children are suboptimal in the United States. In the 2020 to 2021 influenza season, just 58.6% of children aged 6 months to 17 years received at least one dose of influenza vaccine during the season. The youngest children, aged 6 months through 4 years, had the highest influenza vaccination rates (68.0%), whereas older children had lower influenza vaccination rates (5–12 years old 59.0% and 13–17 years old 50.8%).[8] These trends of higher vaccination rates for younger children as compared with older children have persisted during the last decade.[8] There is also wide geographic variation in pediatric influenza vaccination rates. In the 2020 to 2021 influenza season, Mississippi had the lowest influenza vaccination rates at 42.9%, and Massachusetts had the highest rates at 83.6%.[8] Racial/ethnic inequities also persist. For example, among children aged 6 months to 17 years in the 2020 to 2021 influenza season, Asian children had the highest influenza vaccination rates at 69.2%, and American Indian/Alaska Native and Black non-Hispanic children had the lowest rates at 48.3% and 49.1%, respectively. White non-Hispanic children had a vaccination rate of 60.4% followed closely by Hispanic children with a rate of 58.8%. Unfortunately, influenza vaccination rates decreased sharply in the 2020 to 2021 season among children in all age and racial/ethnic groups compared with prior season, and have dropped even further in the 2021 to 2022 season.[8,9] Although there is likely a multitude of reasons for this decline during the COVID-19 pandemic, it does highlight the continued need to address influenza vaccine hesitancy specifically.

Influenza Vaccine Hesitancy

The 15-item Parent Attitudes about Childhood Vaccines (PACV) survey was one of the first tools to be developed and validated to identify parents hesitant about childhood vaccines.[10–12] It has been adapted in multiple languages and short-form versions.[13–18] It also has been modified to assess hesitancy about influenza vaccine.[19–21]

Studies using the PACV survey report that approximately one-quarter of respondents are hesitant about influenza vaccines across different settings. For example, in one single-center study of 152 parents of children presenting to the emergency department in the 2013 to 2014 season, 26% were identified as influenza vaccine hesitant.[21] Similarly, studies conducted among parents of hospitalized children in the 2014 to 2015 (n = 199) and 2017 to 2018 (n = 522) influenza seasons found that 20% and 24%, respectively, were hesitant.[19,20] Parental hesitancy was associated with declination of influenza vaccine for their children in the emergency department and hospital settings.[19–21]

Another commonly used tool to identify vaccine-hesitant individuals is the Vaccine Hesitancy Scale (VHS), which was developed and validated by the World Health Organization's Strategic Advisory Group of Experts on Immunization.[22,23] Similar to the PACV survey, it has been used in diverse populations and settings.[24,25] It has been modified for influenza vaccine.[26] Using the 9-item VHS-Flu Scale, one study found that 26.1% of parents in a nationally representative sample (n = 2052) were hesitant about influenza vaccine, and a lower proportion of hesitant parents had vaccinated their child in the previous season compared with nonhesitant parents (9% vs 76%).[26] Another study conducted in this sample using an 8-item VHS-Flu Scale found that 70% of hesitant parents had ever deferred or refused influenza vaccine for their child due to vaccine concerns compared with 10% of nonhesitant parents.[3] Just as potential inequities exist in receipt of influenza vaccine, certain groups may be more at risk for influenza vaccine hesitancy. Lower education level and household income less than 400% of the federal poverty level were associated with increased influenza vaccine hesitancy.[3] Having more children in the household or being unmarried were also associated with influenza vaccine hesitancy.[3] Conversely, parents who were Hispanic were less hesitant about influenza vaccine than white, non-Hispanic parents.[3]

Impact of the SARS-CoV-2 Pandemic

It remains unclear whether the SARS-CoV-2 pandemic has altered influenza vaccine hesitancy, although the sharp decrease in influenza vaccination rates in children in the 2020 to 2021 season[8] that has continued in 2021 to 2022[9] could reflect some level of increased hesitancy. One survey study conducted in 17 pediatric emergency departments in 6 countries in the spring of 2020 found that, of 1459 caregivers who did not vaccinate their child in the previous season, 70% planned not to vaccinate again in the next season.[27] Similarly, another survey study reported that only 21% of caregivers whose children did not receive the 2019 to 2020 influenza vaccine thought that the pandemic made them more likely to have their child receive the 2020 to 2021 influenza vaccine.[28] Further investigation is needed regarding the impact of the pandemic on parental perspectives and decision-making about influenza vaccination of their children.

Factors that May Impact Influenza Vaccine Hesitancy

To best increase influenza vaccine uptake, one must first understand the myriad factors that can lead to a child either being vaccinated or remaining unvaccinated against influenza. As opposed to other childhood vaccines, influenza vaccine decision-making must occur yearly, meaning that this cycle will replay every year until there is a universal influenza vaccine that can protect people during more than one season.[29]

A useful model for understanding how factors affect vaccination overall and influenza vaccination specifically is the Increasing Vaccination Model from Brewer and colleagues and adapted by the World Health Organization working group.[30] In this model, there are 2 main inputs that lead a family to be "motivated" for their child to be vaccinated: "what people think and feel" and "social processes." Once a family has the motivation to be vaccinated, various "practical issues" can then either facilitate or obstruct the child actually being vaccinated. We have used this model to highlight themes that affect influenza vaccination specifically (**Fig. 1**).

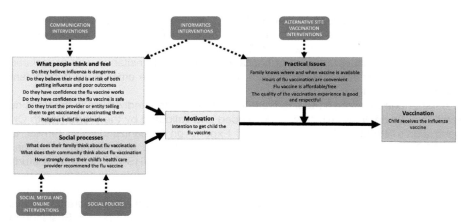

Fig. 1. Using the Increasing Vaccination Model adaptation by World Health Organization working group[29] to understand influenza vaccine hesitancy and potential interventions.

Much research has been conducted trying to understand what people think and feel about influenza and influenza vaccine and how that affects influenza vaccine hesitancy and ultimately influenza vaccination. In its most simplified form, the perceived benefits must outweigh the risks for the parent to decide to vaccinate their child.[31] Families first need to think influenza is dangerous and that their child is at risk of both getting influenza and having a poor outcome.[31–33] Families also need to be confident that the influenza vaccine is effective and that it is safe.[33,34] Compared with other childhood vaccines, parents are less likely to think of influenza vaccines as important for their child's health and less likely to agree that the influenza vaccine is beneficial and a good way to protect their child from influenza.[3] Influenza vaccine effectiveness is complicated. First, it varies from season to season.[35] Second, at its best, seasonal protection against infection ranges between 40% and 60% among the overall population when there is a good match between the strains circulating in a given season and that season's vaccine.[36] Nonetheless, many parents are not aware that the vaccine does avert illness[6] and most importantly that it is effective against severe outcomes from influenza such as intensive care unit hospitalizations and deaths.[37,38] Moreover, some families incorrectly report that their child "caught the flu" after receiving influenza vaccine, not recognizing that many other respiratory illnesses cause influenza-like illnesses and that influenza vaccine cannot prevent those other viral infections.[32]

There are other misperceptions about the influenza vaccine. The most common concern families express is that the influenza vaccine can give people the "flu."[32,39] Although the vaccine cannot cause the "flu," common vaccine side effects can include flu-like symptoms.[35] These perceptions have been shown to negatively affect the intention to vaccinate.[39] Understanding how to communicate with families that influenza vaccines are important and safe, but imperfect, is a critical next step for addressing influenza vaccine hesitancy. Such messaging may also be relevant for COVID-19 vaccine because we move from messaging about protection against any infection to protection against severe outcomes.

Finally, there may be specific knowledge gaps for families of young children aged 6 months through 8 years who need 2 doses in a given season.[34] Receipt of that second dose is very important, and nearly halves the odds of lab-confirmed influenza compared with receipt of only one dose.[40]

Social processes may also affect influenza vaccination. Familial perceptions and experiences regarding influenza vaccination do affect influenza vaccination of children.[41] For example, children are more likely to be vaccinated if their parent was vaccinated as an adult.[42] Community norms regarding influenza vaccination also play a role; families are more likely to vaccinate if they think it is a social norm.[32,33,41,43] Many studies demonstrate that a strong health-care provider recommendation for influenza vaccination positively influences influenza vaccine decision-making.[31,41,43] However, compared with other childhood vaccines, parents are less likely to report following their child's health-care provider recommendations regarding influenza vaccines.[3] Studies have highlighted the importance of a supportive care team working together to encourage influenza vaccination.[44,45] This includes nurses, medical assistants, and front desk staff serving as vaccine champions. In addition, families need to inherently "trust the messenger" who is telling them to get vaccinated or vaccinating them. Distrust of the public health system and/or pharmaceutical companies can erode this process.[46] Religious belief can also play a role in promoting vaccination or increasing vaccine hesitancy.[47] Finally, governmental policies can create external social norms such as when a child's school or day care mandates influenza vaccination bypassing vaccine decision-making by families.[46]

Once a family decides that they do want their child vaccinated then the *practical issues* gain importance. For mildly vaccine-hesitant parents, addressing these practical issues is critical because even small barriers could lead to the child ultimately not being vaccinated. First, a family needs to know where and when influenza vaccine is available. Influenza vaccine is seasonal and not always available at the same point in the fall. Although the Centers for Disease Control and Prevention and American Academy of Pediatrics recommend that children receive their influenza vaccine doses by the end of October,[7] families may often not start to think about vaccination until the mid-fall, leading to a rush to get vaccinated as influenza disease rates increase. Disparities in vaccine supply and delivery may also exist between commercial providers and the Vaccines for Children program,[48] making it even more complicated for families and practices to know when vaccination will begin each season. Families may face barriers to getting the vaccine, such as scheduling an appointment, arranging transportation, or getting time off from work.[31,32] Once a family is at a visit, health-care providers may fail to capture opportunities to vaccinate their patients, particularly during acute care visits.[49,50] Cost of vaccination, although less of a problem at the family level given that it is covered by health insurance as well as the Vaccines for Children program, can be high at a practice level, leading some practices not to stock vaccine.[51] Finally, families need to think they will have a good experience getting vaccinated. Although not specific to the influenza vaccine, we found that families with negative vaccination experiences were more likely to put off a vaccination.[52]

Interventions to Promote Influenza Vaccine Uptake

Knowing influenza vaccine uptake is low and that the factors influencing vaccination are complex, multifaceted interventions that target multiple barriers and challenges, including influenza vaccine hesitancy, are needed.[53–55] Strategies to consider that target aspects of the Intent to Vaccinate Model[30] (see **Fig. 1**) are discussed in detail below.

Influenza Vaccine Communication Strategies to Target what Families Think and Feel

Studies have demonstrated the key role that providers play in parental decision-making about influenza vaccine. For example, a recent study in the pediatric hospital setting revealed that, among parents of vaccine-eligible patients who initially had no plan or planned to decline influenza vaccine during hospitalization, 22% decided to accept the vaccine, and two-thirds of these parents cited a health-care professional (HCP) conversation as the main reason for changing their mind.[45] In that study, a parent-reported HCP vaccine conversation and HCP vaccine recommendation were positively associated with influenza vaccination during hospitalization. Another study of videotaped health supervision visits found that provider use of a presumptive rather than participatory approach to initiating the influenza vaccine recommendation was associated with greater parental acceptance of influenza vaccine for their child, even among vaccine-hesitant families.[56] This study also revealed that other communication strategies, for example, bundling recommendations for influenza and other childhood vaccines and continuing to recommend the vaccine even if families initially declined, were associated with increased influenza vaccine acceptance. A recent study found that scripting in the electronic health record (EHR) to offer a presumptive influenza vaccine recommendation as part of a multifaceted intervention was successful in increasing influenza vaccine administration to hospitalized patients.[57]

Motivational interviewing (MI) may be an effective technique for providers to use when facing initial resistance to their recommendation. A cluster randomized clinical trial of a provider vaccine communication intervention, which included MI training, found that adolescents at intervention practices had higher odds of initiating and completing the human papillomavirus (HPV) vaccine series compared with adolescents at control practices.[58] There are limited data describing the use of MI to address influenza vaccine concerns. However, in a recent pilot study, increased MI competency among physicians addressing influenza vaccine hesitancy in adult patients with rheumatologic disease positively influenced participant attitudes and behaviors related to influenza vaccination.[59]

Finally, there is evidence that having more than one conversation where these communication techniques are used (eg, at separate visits) has a positive influence on childhood vaccination outcomes.[60] Data regarding the dose–response relationship with influenza vaccination are needed. It also may be valuable for multiple members of the care team to communicate about influenza vaccine with families, and consistent messaging across the care team is crucial.[45,61] Learning how best to communicate with parents hesitant about influenza vaccination can be difficult. Immersive virtual reality (VR) is an innovative method to teach influenza vaccine communication skills and facilitate information processing among hesitant patients and families. In an educational study of a VR training curriculum addressing influenza vaccine hesitancy, influenza vaccine refusal rates were lower among patients seen by pediatric residents who underwent the VR training compared with those who did not.[62] More recently, immersive VR has also been used to improve influenza-related perceptions among influenza vaccine-avoidant adult participants.[63]

Interventions to Affect Social Norms

Social media posts and campaigns can influence influenza vaccination decisions. In one social media campaign, researchers paid social media influencers to post prevetted facts about influenza and influenza vaccine on their accounts, which led to improved knowledge and positive attitudes toward influenza vaccine.[64] Another group offered online community health worker-led educational workshops about influenza and influenza vaccine to Latinx families living in underserved communities in Washington state.[65] They also posted on social media, broadcast over radio, developed advertisements, and distributed educational flyers as a supplement. The program improved knowledge about influenza in all participants but was not evaluated for effect on influenza vaccination rates. One university leveraged peer educators to promote influenza vaccine uptake through in-person outreach to students, hanging posters in dormitories, and posting outreach materials on social media, demonstrating substantial improvements in influenza vaccine uptake.[66] Another way to promote influenza vaccine to parents is through advertisements. One group of researchers created and evaluated the effectiveness of online advertisements for influenza, HPV, and zoster vaccines.[67] Results showed that ad viewers who had been searching for vaccine keywords and those who had been searching for unrelated topics were both more likely to click on the ads and search for vaccine-related keywords in the future.[67]

Policies mandating influenza vaccination impose external social norms, leapfrogging vaccine hesitancy concerns, and have been effective in increasing influenza vaccination rates in childcare and preschool settings.[68] Several states require influenza vaccine for childcare and preschool including Connecticut, Massachusetts, New Jersey, New York City (not entire state), Ohio, Pennsylvania, and Rhode Island.[69] A study of New York City's prekindergarten mandate showed that there was a 6.3% to 9.8% increase in influenza vaccination coverage of 4-year-olds in New York City compared with New York state.[70] States may also address vaccine hesitancy by mandating parental counseling by a health-care provider before receiving an exemption to vaccination requirement.[71]

Interventions to Address Practical Issues

One area that has gained prominence during the last few years is the use of informatic tools to promote influenza vaccination, including vaccine-hesitant families who are in the "moveable middle." This is an important group because they are less motivated to be vaccinated and therefore need additional prompts but are not completely against vaccination and therefore can be encouraged to vaccinate given the right information and setting. Text message influenza vaccine reminders have been used by us and other researchers.[72–77] Such reminders have been effective when sent by individual practices, with small but meaningful increases in influenza vaccination. They have, however, not been impactful when being sent by immunization registries,[78] for which an auto-dialer reminder worked better.[79] Text messages tend to be low cost given the ease in which many thousands of people can be sent messages at the same time with extremely low cost per message. Messages can target certain groups or be tailored to make them more personalized. These reminders can help with the practical issues of letting families know when and where vaccine is available. Embedded educational information can also help address different aspects of vaccine hesitancy related to what people may think or feel about influenza vaccine. We have found that for certain populations interactive and embedded educational information in text messages was particularly effective.[73,74] Patient portal messages have been found to be highly effective for receipt of second dose of influenza vaccine for those in need of 2 doses that season but were not effective in the general pediatric population.[80] Some studies in adults have applied behavioral economic messaging such as positive/negative framing, planning prompts, and other psychological messaging innovations to text message or portal reminders with mixed success.[81–83] Several app-based interventions have also been used to improve influenza vaccine uptake, although none have focused on a pediatric population; they have not yet been fully studied for effectiveness in adults.[84–86]

Clinical decision support (CDS) in the EHR is another common informatics tool that can increase influenza vaccine uptake by indirectly targeting vaccine hesitancy. CDS prompts help remind providers and staff to capture opportunities to vaccinate against influenza.[87–89] Similar to text message reminders, they can be used to address what people think and feel by promoting a strong recommendation and tailored communication between the provider and the family. Investigators at Emory found that using a CDS strategy, including a script for offering a presumptive recommendation and information addressing influenza vaccine eligibility, had a positive impact on influenza vaccination rates.[57]

Finally, making it more convenient for families to get influenza vaccine could help those who are mildly hesitant by lowering the activation barrier to have their child be vaccinated. Primary care sites can do this by offering evening or weekend hours for vaccination, as well as remembering to capture opportunities to vaccinate when patients are there for other visits.[90]

Another option for increasing convenience is to offer influenza vaccine in other medical settings outside of primary care such as subspecialty practices, EDs, urgent care centers (UCCs), and hospitals.[91] For example, a survey of UCCs in Arizona showed that one-third offered influenza vaccine to children aged 6 months and older.[92] Most pediatricians are in favor of influenza vaccination in schools or other settings within the community, especially for healthy school-aged children.[93] Offering influenza vaccination in schools, that is, at school-based health centers or in partnership with local departments of health that host temporary vaccine clinics within the school, is one evidence-based way to improve childhood influenza vaccination rates.[94–98] For example, one randomized control trial involving 44 schools in New York demonstrated that school-located influenza vaccine clinics improved coverage in both suburban and urban settings and did not displace vaccination at primary care sites in the suburban setting.[98] Pharmacies can also help improve influenza vaccination coverage in communities. Laws authorizing pharmacists to provide vaccinations to children, including influenza vaccine, differ by state but had been expanding even before the COVID-19 pandemic.[99] One study conducted among pharmacies in Oregon found that influenza vaccination of adolescents increased at pharmacies but did not decline at other places suggesting that pharmacies were reaching adolescents who may not have otherwise gone to their doctor for vaccination.[100] Finally, collaboration with community-based organizations, churches, and other sites has been helpful for adult influenza vaccination[101] but is not commonly reported in pediatric or adolescent populations.

Regardless of where influenza vaccine is given, a clear and consistent message about its benefits as well as the ability to address vaccine concerns with potentially hesitant families is needed. It is also crucial that entities report vaccine administrations to their local Immunization Information System (IIS)[102] so that accurate, complete, vaccine information is readily accessible across providers and locations.[103] As more children and adolescents are vaccinating in alternative sites, IIS integration with EHRs could further reduce over/undervaccination.[104]

SUMMARY

Although influenza vaccine coverage is suboptimal, even small incremental increases in influenza vaccination can have important health impacts. The CDC estimates that a 5% increase in national influenza vaccination coverage could prevent 228,000 illnesses and 4900 hospitalizations across all age groups during seasons with typical influenza severity.[105] Multilevel strategies are needed to improve uptake. Particular emphasis on addressing influenza vaccine hesitancy is crucial given the higher level of hesitancy that exists for influenza vaccine as compared with other childhood vaccines.[3] Importantly, we need parents to understand that influenza can be serious, that their child is at risk of influenza, and that the influenza vaccine is safe, cannot cause "the flu," and will help protect them, particularly from serious outcomes. Influenza vaccine providers across diverse settings must use effective communication techniques because they discuss influenza and influenza vaccine and quell false beliefs that patients and families may have. This includes using a strong, consistent, and presumptive recommendation for annual influenza vaccination as well as clear messaging about the benefits of influenza vaccination. Efforts in the health-care settings could be augmented by EHR-embedded CDS, prompting providers to recommend influenza vaccine for patients who are due and giving them evidence-based scripts for talking with families. Practices can also be encouraged to use reminders for influenza vaccination, including those that embed educational information to target vaccine hesitancy. It is also crucial to increase access to influenza vaccination by expanding opportunities to receive vaccine at primary care offices as well as at other health-care settings, schools, community events, and other nontraditional venues. This will make it easier and more convenient for families to vaccinate their children. Finally, we need to focus on ways to promote annual influenza vaccination as a social norm, which may help those who are mildly hesitant. Efforts to change attitudes and beliefs may be aided by outreach campaigns via social media, advertisements, or other means to help normalize influenza vaccination and make it more widely accepted in one's family, community, and social sphere.

Overall, although each of these actions might individually have small effects, together they will hopefully move the needle on influenza vaccine hesitancy and increase national influenza vaccination coverage. Even very small increases can save lives.

CLINICS CARE POINTS

- Particular characteristics of influenza vaccine make it more prone to hesitancy, including that influenza vaccine effectiveness is lower than that of other vaccines, the vaccine is required annually, and there are specific false beliefs related to it.

- The PACV and VHS are 2 evidence-based tools that can measure influenza vaccine hesitancy.

- Evidence-based strategies such as a strong, presumptive, provider recommendation of influenza vaccine, CDS in the EMR, text message and vaccine reminder/recall including via text messaging can help promote influenza vaccination, potentially in part by overcoming influenza vaccine hesitancy.

FINANCIAL DISCLOSURE

No financial disclosures were reported by the authors of this article.

FUNDING

M.S. Stockwell reports research funding from the Centers for Disease Control and Prevention and the National Institutes of Health.

CONFLICTS OF INTEREST

The authors have no conflicts of interest to report.

REFERENCES

1. Victorian Health Reform. Available at. https://www.nationalarchives.gov.uk/education/resources/victorian-health-reform/. Accessed on May 10, 2022.

2. Spier RE. Perception of risk of vaccine adverse events: a historical perspective. Vaccine 2001;20:S78–84.

3. Kempe A, Saville AW, Albertin C, et al. Parental hesitancy about routine childhood and influenza vaccinations: a national survey. Pediatrics 2020;146(1).

4. Centers for Disease Control and Prevention. Influenza Historic Timeline. Available at. https://www.cdc.gov/flu/pandemic-resources/pandemic-timeline-1930-and-beyond.htm. Accessed on May 31, 2022.

5. Schmid P, Rauber D, Betsch C, et al. Barriers of Influenza Vaccination Intention and Behavior - A Systematic Review of Influenza Vaccine Hesitancy, 2005 - 2016. PLoS One 2017;12(1):e0170550.

6. Rolfes MA, Flannery B, Chung JR, et al. Effects of Influenza Vaccination in the United States During the 2017-2018 Influenza Season. Clin Infect Dis 2019; 69(11):1845–53.

7. Grohskopf LA, Alyanak E, Ferdinands JM, et al. Prevention and Control of Seasonal Influenza with Vaccines: Recommendations of the Advisory Committee on Immunization Practices, United States, 2021-22 Influenza Season. MMWR Recomm Rep 2021;70(5):1–28.

8. Centers for Disease Control and Prevention. Flu Vaccination Coverage, United States, 2020–21 Influenza Season. Available at. https://www.cdc.gov/flu/fluvaxview/coverage-2021estimates.htm. Accessed on April 14, 2022.

9. Centers for Disease Control and Prevention. Weekly Flu Vaccination Dashboard. Available at. https://www.cdc.gov/flu/fluvaxview/dashboard/vaccination-dashboard.html. Accessed on July 24, 2022.

10. Opel DJ, Mangione-Smith R, Taylor JA, et al. Development of a survey to identify vaccine-hesitant parents: the parent attitudes about childhood vaccines survey. Hum Vaccin 2011;7(4):419–25.

11. Opel DJ, Taylor JA, Mangione-Smith R, et al. Validity and reliability of a survey to identify vaccine-hesitant parents. Vaccine 2011;29(38):6598–605.

12. Opel DJ, Taylor JA, Zhou C, et al. The relationship between parent attitudes about childhood vaccines survey scores and future child immunization status: a validation study. JAMA Pediatr 2013;167(11):1065–71.

13. Abd Halim H, Abdul-Razak S, Md Yasin M, et al. Validation study of the Parent Attitudes About Childhood Vaccines (PACV) questionnaire: the Malay version. Hum Vaccin Immunother 2020;16(5):1040–9.

14. Alsuwaidi AR, Elbarazi I, Al-Hamad S, et al. Vaccine hesitancy and its determinants among Arab parents: a cross-sectional survey in the United Arab Emirates. Hum Vaccin Immunother 2020;16(12):3163–9.

15. Cunningham RM, Kerr GB, Orobio J, et al. Development of a Spanish version of the parent attitudes about childhood vaccines survey. Hum Vaccin Immunother 2019;15(5):1106–10.

16. Oladejo O, Allen K, Amin A, et al. Comparative analysis of the Parent Attitudes about Childhood Vaccines (PACV) short scale and the five categories of vaccine acceptance identified by Gust et al. Vaccine 2016;34(41):4964–8.

17. Olarewaju VO, Jafflin K, Deml MJ, et al. Application of the Parent Attitudes about Childhood Vaccines (PACV) survey in three national languages in Switzerland: Exploratory factor analysis and Mokken scale analysis. Hum Vaccin Immunother 2021;17(8):2652–60.

18. Opel DJ, Henrikson N, Lepere K, et al. Previsit screening for parental vaccine hesitancy: a cluster randomized trial. Pediatrics 2019;144(5).

19. Hofstetter AM, Opel DJ, Stockwell MS, et al. Influenza-related knowledge, beliefs, and experiences among caregivers of hospitalized children. Hosp Pediatr 2021;11(8):815–32.
20. Hofstetter AM, Simon TD, Lepere K, et al. Parental vaccine hesitancy and declination of influenza vaccination among hospitalized children. Hosp Pediatr 2018; 8(10):628–35.
21. Strelitz B, Gritton J, Klein EJ, et al. Parental vaccine hesitancy and acceptance of seasonal influenza vaccine in the pediatric emergency department. Vaccine 2015;33(15):1802–7.
22. Larson HJ, Jarrett C, Schulz WS, et al. Measuring vaccine hesitancy: The development of a survey tool. Vaccine 2015;33(34):4165–75.
23. Shapiro GK, Tatar O, Dube E, et al. The vaccine hesitancy scale: Psychometric properties and validation. Vaccine 2018;36(5):660–7.
24. Domek GJ, O'Leary ST, Bull S, et al. Measuring vaccine hesitancy: Field testing the WHO SAGE Working Group on Vaccine Hesitancy survey tool in Guatemala. Vaccine 2018;36(35):5273–81.
25. Gentile A, Pacchiotti AC, Giglio N, et al. Vaccine hesitancy in Argentina: Validation of WHO scale for parents. Vaccine 2021;39(33):4611–9.
26. Helmkamp LJ, Szilagyi PG, Zimet G, et al. A validated modification of the vaccine hesitancy scale for childhood, influenza and HPV vaccines. Vaccine 2021; 39(13):1831–9.
27. Goldman RD, McGregor S, Marneni SR, et al. Willingness to Vaccinate Children against Influenza after the Coronavirus Disease 2019 Pandemic. J Pediatr 2021; 228:87–93 e82.
28. Sokol RL, Grummon AH. COVID-19 and Parent Intention to Vaccinate Their Children Against Influenza. Pediatrics 2020;146(6).
29. Estrada LD, Schultz-Cherry S. Development of a Universal Influenza Vaccine. J Immunol 2019;202(2):392–8.
30. Brewer NT. What Works to Increase Vaccination Uptake. Acad Pediatr 2021; 21(4S):S9–16.
31. Malosh R, Ohmit SE, Petrie JG, et al. Factors associated with influenza vaccine receipt in community dwelling adults and their children. Vaccine 2014;32(16): 1841–7.
32. Flood EM, Rousculp MD, Ryan KJ, et al. Parents' decision-making regarding vaccinating their children against influenza: A web-based survey. Clin Ther 2010;32(8):1448–67.
33. Allison MA, Reyes M, Young P, et al. Parental attitudes about influenza immunization and school-based immunization for school-aged children. Pediatr Infect Dis J 2010;29(8):751–5.
34. Hofstetter AM, Barrett A, Stockwell MS. Factors impacting influenza vaccination of urban low-income Latino children under nine years requiring two doses in the 2010-2011 season. J Community Health 2015;40(2):227–34.
35. Centers for Disease Control and Prevention. Misconceptions about Seasonal Flu and Flu Vaccines. Available at. https://www.cdc.gov/flu/prevent/misconceptions.htm. Accessed on June 3, 2022.
36. Centers for Disease Control and Prevention. Vaccine Effectiveness: How Well Do Flu Vaccines Work?. Available at. https://www.cdc.gov/flu/vaccines-work/vaccineeffect.htm. Accessed on May 4, 2022.
37. Ferdinands JM, Olsho LE, Agan AA, et al. Effectiveness of influenza vaccine against life-threatening RT-PCR-confirmed influenza illness in US children, 2010-2012. J Infect Dis 2014;210(5):674–83.

38. Flannery B, Reynolds SB, Blanton L, et al. Influenza vaccine effectiveness against pediatric deaths: 2010-2014. Pediatrics 2017;139(5).

39. Grant VJ, Le Saux N, Plint AC, et al. Factors influencing childhood influenza immunization. CMAJ 2003;168(1):39–41.

40. Chung JR, Flannery B, Gaglani M, et al. Patterns of Influenza Vaccination and Vaccine Effectiveness Among Young US Children Who Receive Outpatient Care for Acute Respiratory Tract Illness. JAMA Pediatr 2020;174(7):705–13.

41. Lin CJ, Zimmerman RK, Nowalk MP, et al. Parental perspectives on influenza vaccination of children with chronic medical conditions. J Natl Med Assoc 2006;98(2):148–53.

42. Goss MD, Temte JL, Barlow S, et al. An assessment of parental knowledge, attitudes, and beliefs regarding influenza vaccination. Vaccine 2020;38(6): 1565–71.

43. Daley MF, Crane LA, Chandramouli V, et al. Influenza among healthy young children: changes in parental attitudes and predictors of immunization during the 2003 to 2004 influenza season. Pediatrics 2006;117(2):e268–77.

44. Nowalk MP, Lin CJ, Zimmerman RK, et al. Tailored interventions to introduce influenza vaccination among 6- to 23-month-old children at inner-city health centers. Am J Manag Care 2005;11(11):717–24.

45. Hofstetter AM, Opel DJ, Stockwell MS, et al. Associations between health care professional communication practices and influenza vaccination of hospitalized children. Acad Pediatr 2021;21(7):1142–50.

46. Bhat-Schelbert K, Lin CJ, Matambanadzo A, et al. Barriers to and facilitators of child influenza vaccine - perspectives from parents, teens, marketing and healthcare professionals. Vaccine 2012;30(14):2448–52.

47. Green HK, Andrews N, Letley L, et al. Phased introduction of a universal childhood influenza vaccination programme in England: population-level factors predicting variation in national uptake during the first year, 2013/14. Vaccine 2015; 33(22):2620–8.

48. Bhatt P, Block SL, Toback SL, et al. Timing of the availability and administration of influenza vaccine through the vaccines for children program. Pediatr Infect Dis J 2011;30(2):100–6.

49. Verani JR, Irigoyen M, Chen S, et al. Influenza vaccine coverage and missed opportunities among inner-city children aged 6 to 23 months: 2000-2005. Pediatrics 2007;119(3):e580–6.

50. Dombkowski KJ, Davis MM, Cohn LM, et al. Effect of missed opportunities on influenza vaccination rates among children with asthma. Arch Pediatr Adolesc Med 2006;160(9):966–71.

51. Yoo BK, Szilagyi PG, Schaffer SJ, et al. Cost of universal influenza vaccination of children in pediatric practices. Pediatrics 2009;124(Suppl 5):S499–506.

52. Stockwell MS, Irigoyen M, Andres Martinez R, et al. Failure to return: parental, practice, and social factors affecting missed immunization visits for urban children. Clin Pediatr (Phila) 2014;53(5):420–7.

53. Fiks AG, Nekrasova E, Hambidge SJ. Health Systems as a Catalyst for Immunization Delivery. Acad Pediatr 2021;21(4S):S40–7.

54. Stockwell MS, Stokley S, Kempe A. Implementing Effective Vaccination Interventions Into Sustainable 'Real World' Practice. Acad Pediatr 2021;21(4S):S78–80.

55. Stokley S, Kempe A, Stockwell MS, et al. Improving Pediatric Vaccination Coverage in the United States. Acad Pediatr 2021;21(4S):S1–2.

56. Hofstetter AM, Robinson JD, Lepere K, et al. Clinician-parent discussions about influenza vaccination of children and their association with vaccine acceptance. Vaccine 2017;35(20):2709–15.

57. Orenstein EW, ElSayed-Ali O, Kandaswamy S, et al. Evaluation of a Clinical Decision Support Strategy to Increase Seasonal Influenza Vaccination Among Hospitalized Children Before Inpatient Discharge. JAMA Netw Open 2021;4(7): e2117809.

58. Dempsey AF, Pyrznawoski J, Lockhart S, et al. Effect of a Health Care Professional Communication Training Intervention on Adolescent Human Papillomavirus Vaccination: A Cluster Randomized Clinical Trial. JAMA Pediatr 2018; 172(5):e180016.

59. Labbe S, Colmegna I, Valerio V, et al. Training Physicians in Motivational Communication to Address Influenza Vaccine Hesitation: A Proof-of-Concept Study. Vaccines (Basel) 2022;10(2).

60. Opel DJ, Zhou C, Robinson JD, et al. Impact of Childhood Vaccine Discussion Format Over Time on Immunization Status. Acad Pediatr 2018;18(4):430–6.

61. Fontenot HB, Kornides ML, McRee AL, et al. Importance of a team approach to recommending the human papillomavirus vaccination. J Am Assoc Nurse Pract 2018;30(7):368–72.

62. Real FJ, DeBlasio D, Beck AF, et al. A Virtual Reality Curriculum for Pediatric Residents Decreases Rates of Influenza Vaccine Refusal. Acad Pediatr 2017; 17(4):431–5.

63. Nowak GJ, Evans NJ, Wojdynski BW, et al. Using immersive virtual reality to improve the beliefs and intentions of influenza vaccine avoidant 18-to-49-year-olds: Considerations, effects, and lessons learned. Vaccine 2020;38(5): 1225–33.

64. Bonnevie E, Rosenberg SD, Kummeth C, et al. Using social media influencers to increase knowledge and positive attitudes toward the flu vaccine. PLoS One 2020;15(10):e0240828.

65. Ponce-Gonzalez IM, Perez K, Cheadle AD, et al. A multicomponent health education campaign led by community health workers to increase influenza vaccination among migrants and refugees. J Prim Care Community Health 2021;12. 21501327211055627.

66. Huang JA-O, Francesconi M, Cooper MH, et al. Community health workers on a college campus: Effects on influenza vaccination. J Am Coll Health 2018;66(4): 317–23.

67. Krupenkin M, Yom-Tov EA-O, Rothschild D. Vaccine advertising: preach to the converted or to the unaware? NPJ Digit Med 2021;4(1):23.

68. Hadler JL, Yousey-Hindes K, Kudish K, et al. Impact of requiring influenza vaccination for children in licensed child care or preschool programs–Connecticut, 2012-13 influenza season. MMWR Morb Mortal Wkly Rep 2014;63(9):181–5.

69. Influenza Vaccine Mandates for Child Care and Pre-K. Available at. https://www.immunize.org/laws/flu_childcare.asp. Accessed on April 15, 2022.

70. Hong K, Lindley MC, Tsai Y, et al. School Mandate and Influenza Vaccine Uptake Among Prekindergartners in New York City, 2012-2019. Am J Public Health 2022;112(5):719–23.

71. Omer SB, Allen K, Chang DH, et al. Exemptions From Mandatory Immunization After Legally Mandated Parental Counseling. Pediatrics 2018;141(1).

72. Stockwell MS, Kharbanda EO, Martinez RA, et al. Effect of a text messaging intervention on influenza vaccination in an urban, low-income pediatric and

adolescent population: a randomized controlled trial. JAMA 2012;307(16): 1702–8.

73. Stockwell MS, Hofstetter AM, DuRivage N, et al. Text message reminders for second dose of influenza vaccine: a randomized controlled trial. Pediatrics 2015;135(1):e83–91.

74. Hofstetter AM, Vargas CY, Camargo S, et al. Impacting delayed pediatric influenza vaccination: a randomized controlled trial of text message reminders. Am J Prev Med 2015;48(4):392–401.

75. Hofstetter AM, Barrett A, Camargo S, et al. Text message reminders for vaccination of adolescents with chronic medical conditions: A randomized clinical trial. Vaccine 2017;35(35 Pt B):4554–60.

76. Sloand E, VanGraafeiland B, Holm A, et al. Text message quality improvement project for influenza vaccine in a low-resource largely latino pediatric population. J Healthc Qual 2019;41(6):362–8.

77. Jacobson Vann JC, Jacobson RM, Coyne-Beasley T, et al. Patient reminder and recall interventions to improve immunization rates. Cochrane Database Syst Rev 2018;1:CD003941.

78. Szilagyi PG, Albertin CS, Saville AW, et al. Effect of state immunization information system based reminder/recall for influenza vaccinations: a randomized trial of autodialer, text, and mailed messages. J Pediatr 2020;221:123–131 e124.

79. Kempe A, Saville AW, Albertin C, et al. Centralized reminder/recall to increase influenza vaccination rates: a two-state pragmatic randomized trial. Acad Pediatr 2020;20(3):374–83.

80. Lerner C, Albertin C, Casillas A, et al. Patient portal reminders for pediatric influenza vaccinations: a randomized clinical trial. Pediatrics 2021;148(2).

81. Milkman KL, Patel MS, Gandhi L, et al. A megastudy of text-based nudges encouraging patients to get vaccinated at an upcoming doctor's appointment. Proc Natl Acad Sci U S A 2021;118(20).

82. Buttenheim A, Milkman KL, Duckworth AL, et al. Effects of ownership text message wording and reminders on receipt of an influenza vaccination: a randomized clinical trial. JAMA Netw Open 2022;5(2):e2143388.

83. Szilagyi PG, Albertin CS, Casillas A, et al. Effect of Personalized Messages Sent by a Health System's Patient Portal on Influenza Vaccination Rates: a Randomized Clinical Trial. J Gen Intern Med 2022;37(3):615–23.

84. Lee W-N, Stück D, Konty K, et al. Large-scale influenza vaccination promotion on a mobile app platform: A randomized controlled trial. Vaccine 2020;38(18): 3508–14.

85. Salmon DA, Limaye RJ, Dudley MZ, et al. MomsTalkShots: An individually tailored educational application for maternal and infant vaccines. Vaccine 2019;37(43):6478–85.

86. Dale LP, White L, Mitchell M, et al. Smartphone app uses loyalty point incentives and push notifications to encourage influenza vaccine uptake. Vaccine 2019; 37(32):4594–600.

87. Stockwell MS, Catallozzi M, Camargo S, et al. Registry-linked electronic influenza vaccine provider reminders: a cluster-crossover trial. Pediatrics 2015; 135(1):e75–82.

88. Fiks AG, Grundmeier RW, Biggs LM, et al. Impact of clinical alerts within an electronic health record on routine childhood immunization in an urban pediatric population. Pediatrics 2007;120(4):707–14.

89. Au L, Oster A, Yeh GH, et al. Utilizing an electronic health record system to improve vaccination coverage in children. Appl Clin Inform 2010;1(3):221–31.

90. Committee On Infectious Diseases. Recommendations for prevention and control of influenza in children, 2021-2022. Pediatrics 2021;148(4). e2021053745.
91. Hofstetter AM, Schaffer S. Childhood and adolescent vaccination in alternative settings. Acad Pediatr 2021;21(4S):S50–6.
92. Beatty NL, Hager KM, McKeown KR, et al. Influenza vaccine availability at urgent care centers in the state of Arizona. Am J Infect Control 2018;46(8):946–8.
93. Kempe A, Wortley P, O'Leary S, et al. Pediatricians' attitudes about collaborations with other community vaccinators in the delivery of seasonal influenza vaccine. Acad Pediatr 2012;12(1):26–35.
94. Benjamin-Chung J, Arnold BF, Kennedy CJ, et al. Evaluation of a city-wide school-located influenza vaccination program in Oakland, California, with respect to vaccination coverage, school absences, and laboratory-confirmed influenza: A matched cohort study. Plos Med 2020;17(8):e1003238.
95. Pannaraj PS, Wang H-L, Rivas H, et al. School-located influenza vaccination decreases laboratory-confirmed influenza and improves school attendance. Clin Infect 2014;59(3):325–32.
96. Szilagyi PA-O, Schaffer S, Rand CM, et al. School-Located Influenza Vaccination: Do Vaccine Clinics at School Raise Vaccination Rates? J Sch Health 2019;89(12):1004–12.
97. Tran CH, Sugimoto JD, Pulliam JRC, et al. School-located influenza vaccination reduces community risk for influenza and influenza-like illness emergency care visits. PLoS One 2014;9(12):e114479.
98. Szilagyi PG, Schaffer S, Rand CM, et al. School-Located Influenza Vaccinations: A Randomized Trial. Pediatrics 2016;138(5).
99. Schmit CD, Penn MS. Expanding state laws and a growing role for pharmacists in vaccination services. J Am Pharm Assoc (2003) 2017;57(6):661–9.
100. Robison SG. Impact of pharmacists providing immunizations on adolescent influenza immunization. J Am Pharm Assoc (2003) 2016;56(4):446–9.
101. Mosesso VN Jr, Packer R, McMahon J, et al. Influenze immunizations provided by EMS agencies: The MEDICVAX project. Prehosp Emerg Care 2003;7(1):74.
102. Centers for Disease Control and Prevention. Progress in immunization information systems - United States, 2012. MMWR Morb Mortal Wkly Rep 2013;62(49):1005–8.
103. Birmingham E, Catallozzi M, Findley SE, et al. FluAlert: a qualitative evaluation of providers' desired characteristics and concerns regarding computerized influenza vaccination alerts. Prev Med 2011;52(3–4):274–7.
104. Stockwell MS, Natarajan K, Ramakrishnan R, et al. Immunization data exchange with electronic health records. Pediatrics 2016;137(6).
105. Hughes MM, Reed C, Flannery B, et al. Projected population benefit of increased effectiveness and coverage of influenza vaccination on influenza burden in the United States. Clin Infect Dis 2020;70(12):2496–502.

Coronavirus Disease-2019 Vaccine Hesitancy

E. Adrianne Hammershaimb, MD[a,b], James D. Campbell, MD[a,b],
Sean T. O'Leary, MD, MPH[c,*]

KEYWORDS

- COVID-19 • SARS-CoV-2 • Vaccine • Vaccination • Pediatric • Children
- Vaccine hesitancy • Pandemic

KEY POINTS

- Reluctance around coronavirus disease-2019 (COVID-19) vaccines is associated with unique concerns about their novelty and safety.
- Parents weighing the risks of COVID-19 disease against the risks of COVID-19 vaccination may make different decisions for themselves versus their children.
- Although COVID-19 vaccines have been highly politicized and subject to public scrutiny, pediatricians remain a trusted source of information and guidance.

INTRODUCTION

On December 30, 2019, the World Health Organization (WHO) announced the emergence of severe acute respiratory syndrome coronavirus 2 (SARS-CoV-2) as a novel human pathogen and the causative agent of coronavirus disease 2019 (COVID-19).[1] The pathogen quickly spread across the globe, resulting in a pandemic that caused more than half a billion cases and 6 million deaths by June 2022.[2] Efforts to develop a vaccine were promptly launched with the United States, UK, China, Russia, and India leading the race. COVID-19 vaccines were developed and authorized for use in Russia by August 11, 2020, the UK by December 2, 2020, the United States by December 11, 2020, and China by December 30, 2020.[3–6] It was estimated early on that 70% of the population would need to be vaccinated to end the pandemic; however, hesitancy around COVID-19 vaccines has proven a formidable obstacle to

[a] Division of Infectious Diseases and Tropical Pediatrics, Department of Pediatrics, University of Maryland School of Medicine, Baltimore, MD, USA; [b] Center for Vaccine Development and Global Health, University of Maryland, School of Medicine, Health Sciences Research Facility 1, Research Facility 1, Room 480, 685 West Baltimore Street, Baltimore, MD 21201, USA; [c] Department of Pediatrics, University of Colorado Anschutz Medical Campus, F443, 1890 North Revere Court, Aurora, CO 80045, USA
* Corresponding author. Adult and Child Center for Health Outcomes Research and Delivery Science, University of Colorado Anschutz Medical Campus and Children's Hospital Colorado, F443, 1890 North Revere Court, Aurora, CO 80045.
E-mail address: SEAN.OLEARY@CUANSCHUTZ.EDU

Pediatr Clin N Am 70 (2023) 243–257
https://doi.org/10.1016/j.pcl.2022.12.001
0031-3955/23/© 2022 Elsevier Inc. All rights reserved.
pediatric.theclinics.com

achieving target vaccination levels.[7] Understanding the factors related to COVID-19 vaccine acceptance vs. reluctance/refusal would be an integral component of eventual vaccination campaigns, theoretically providing opportunities to bolster acceptance and mitigate hesitancy.

Early in the pandemic, before COVID-19 vaccines were authorized and disseminated, public opinion polls began tracking public acceptance of and concerns about a hypothetical COVID-19 vaccine. Over time, as vaccines and information about them have become more widely available, the focus has shifted from evaluating premeditative thoughts about COVID-19 vaccines to observing behaviors, measuring vaccine uptake, and characterizing factors associated with COVID-19 vaccine acceptance. Much of what was initially understood about public opinions of COVID-19 vaccines was both garnered by and shared through the lay media. Throughout the pandemic, a wealth of peer-reviewed literature examining the complexities of COVID-19 vaccine acceptance has also emerged, but our understanding of COVID-19 vaccine acceptance is constantly evolving along with the pandemic itself.

CORONAVIRUS DISEASE-2019 VACCINE INTENTIONS BEFORE AUTHORIZATION

During the initial wave of the pandemic in North America and Western Europe, public opinion was largely supportive of vaccines against COVID-19. A large survey across 19 countries in June 2020 found that willingness to take a COVID-19 once available was 72% worldwide and as high as 76% and 75% in Mexico and the United States, respectively, and 69% in Canada.[8] By September 2020, at the height of a US presidential election campaign season, President Trump was promising an FDA-approved vaccine ahead of election day. At that time acceptance had dropped to as low as 63% in the general US population with only 34% saying they would "definitely get" a COVID-19 vaccine "if it were free and deemed safe by scientists."[9]

CORONAVIRUS DISEASE-2019 VACCINE INTENTIONS AND UPTAKE DURING ROLLOUTS
Adult Rollout

After the US Food and Drug Administration (FDA) authorized the first COVID-19 vaccines for use in the United States, initial guidance from the Centers for Diseases Control and Prevention (CDC) Advisory Committee on Immunization Practices (ACIP) prioritized residents of long-term care facilities (LTCFs), due to the high rates of morbidity and mortality in this population, and health care workers (HCWs), due to concerns about the strain on the health care system.[10] In the first month of the US COVID-19 vaccine rollout, HCW uptake was generally high. Although receipt was also high (78%) LTCF residents only 38% of LTCF staff members had received one or more doses of a COVID-19 vaccine through the CDC Pharmacy Partnership for Long-Term Care Program.[11] By April 2021, vaccination among health care providers working in LTCFs had increased to 57% with the highest rates among physicians and advanced practice providers (75%) and lower rates among nurses and ancillary services employees (57% and 59%, respectively).[12] Lower rates of vaccine acceptance among nurses relative to physicians have been noted in health care systems across the United States, Canada, and internationally.[13–18] Other characteristics of HCWs associated with decreased acceptance include younger age, female sex, Black race, and Hispanic/Latino ethnicity. These were similar to characteristics associated with decreased acceptance found in the general US population at that time.[17–19]

Other frontline workers, older adults, and people with chronic medical conditions were also prioritized for early vaccination. Compared with healthy adults, those with chronic medical conditions, including immunocompromising conditions, were more accepting of COVID-19 vaccination, and the perception of being at increased risk of severe COVID-19 disease was associated with increased acceptance.[20–22] In contrast, a December 2020 survey found that 35% of US essential workers were not likely to get a COVID-19 vaccine.[22] By mid-March 2021%, 48% of non-health care essential workers in the United States had received a COVID-19 vaccine with 21% still reporting they would not get one, even if required.[23]

Following the authorization of COVID-19 vaccines, surveys conducted in January 2021 showed that 47% of US adults were either vaccinated or intended to get a COVID-19 vaccine as soon as one became available to them, whereas 72% of Canadian adults intended to get a COVID-19 vaccine.[24,25] Over the subsequent months with increasing access to vaccines, uptake among US adults increased with 62% reporting that they had received a COVID-19 vaccine by May 2021.[24] Uptake among adults 65 years and older has been quite high in the United States and Canada (Mexico does not breakdown vaccination data by age). For example, in the US, as of July 29%, 2022%, 92% of adults 65 and older are fully vaccinated, although there is a great deal of geographic variability at the state and county levels.[26]

Pediatric Rollout

In the United States, the Pfizer/BioNTech COVID-19 vaccine had been authorized for adolescents 16 years and older since December 2020, and in May 2021, the vaccine was authorized for adolescents 12 to 15 years of age. By the end of July 2021%, 43% of US adolescents 12 to 17 years old had received a COVID-19 vaccine with subsequent slow increases to a plateau of approximately 68% by February 2022. This trajectory is consistent with surveys showing that one-third of US parents wanted to "wait and see" before vaccinating their children.[24,27–29] In October-November 2021, similar proportions of US parents of 5- to 11-year-old children reported wanting to wait before vaccinating their children, with 22% to 27% wanting to vaccinate them as soon as possible.[24,30] A vaccine was authorized for children 5 to 11 years old in the United States on October 29, 2021, and by the end of January 2022%, 31% of US children 5 to 11 years old had received at least a first dose of COVID-19 vaccine. However, as of July 2022%, 63% of US children in this age group remain completely unvaccinated.[27,28] As with the adult COVID-19 vaccine rollout, there is wide geographic variation in uptake.[26]

In December 2020%, 63% of Canadian parents intended to vaccinate their children 0 to 17 years of age, and by May 8%, 2022%, 57% and 88% of Canadians 5 to 11 and 12 to 17 years, respectively, had received a COVID-19 vaccine.[31,32] On June 17, 2022, the US FDA authorized COVID-19 vaccines for use in children 6 months-4 years of age, and as of this writing, the rollout of vaccines for children under 5 years was newly underway.[33]

There are limited data on vaccine attitudes among parents of Mexican children.[34] Mexico delayed its vaccination campaign for children, only beginning to vaccinate children 12 years and older with comorbidities after a court order to do so in November 2021, starting with adolescents 15 to 17 years of age.[35] On April 28, 2022, vaccination began for all children 12 and older and Mexico didn't authorize vaccination of 5- to 11-year-olds until May 27, 2022.[26]

CORONAVIRUS DISEASE-2019 VACCINE INCENTIVES AND MANDATES

Efforts to increase vaccine uptake among the general population included both monetary incentives and mandates tied to education, work, entertainment, and travel. Such mandates have been politically contentious and variably effective. A large survey found that cash incentives such as gift cards and entry into lotteries would have no effect on the intentions of roughly half of unvaccinated US adults and would make 40% of those who were disinclined to get a COVID-19 vaccine even less likely to get one.[36] The same survey found that 64% of those unvaccinated Americans who were not inclined to get a COVID-19 vaccine would not get one despite workplace requirements.[36] Despite opinion surveys suggesting that mandates may not be effective and vocal protests and legal actions against vaccine mandates, many entities, including corporations, colleges and universities, health care systems, and government agencies including the military saw significant increases in the numbers of vaccinated employees and students after the introduction of COVID-19 vaccine mandates.[37] For example, Tyson Foods saw an increase in employee vaccinations from 50% to 96% within 3 months of instituting a vaccine mandate, with "very few" employees leaving the company.[38]

SPECIAL POPULATIONS
Black and Hispanic Communities

Black and Latino/Hispanic communities in the United States have experienced disproportionately high rates of morbidity and mortality due to COVID-19 but in general were late adopters of COVID-19 vaccines.[27,39,40] Early reluctance to receive a COVID-19 vaccine was attributed to a mistrust of government and American medicine given personal experiences and a history of abuses by the medical community.[41–43] Data from the CDC's National Immunization Survey – Adult COVID Module (NIS-ACM), which is based on self-report, suggest that the rates of Black, non-Hispanic and Hispanic Americans who have received a COVID-19 vaccine caught up to the rates of vaccinated White, non-Hispanic Americans by October 2021.[27] However, using other data sources on vaccine administration, as of July 29, 2022, vaccination rates among Black, non-Hispanic Americans seem to continue to lag behind those of all other racial and ethnic categories. Similarly, other than Black, and Non-Hispanic Americans, all other racial and ethnic categories have outpaced White, and Non-Hispanic Americans in COVID-19 vaccine uptake.[27] These vaccine administration data, however, are limited in that race and ethnicity are missing for a large portion of the population. This inconsistency between self-reported vaccination status and vaccine administration data highlights the challenge of collecting and reporting accurate data on vaccine-related attitudes and behaviors among different racial and ethnic groups.

Detained Populations

Congregate living settings were the foci of early outbreaks; however, residents of detention centers in the United States were not consistently prioritized in the way that residents of LTCFs were despite recommendations from CDC's ACIP. However, limited access is not the only determinant of COVID-19 vaccine uptake in this population.[44] Studies in the United States and Canada found that incarcerated individuals reported their significant reasons for refusing COVID-19 vaccination to include (1) distrust of prison employees, including HCWs, and the government, and (2) perceiving themselves to be at low risk of COVID-19 disease.[45–47] Similar data on Mexico and other Central American countries are not available as of this writing.[48]

Pregnant Persons

Pregnant persons were largely excluded from the early vaccine trials. Consequently, early prioritization schemes offered little guidance around COVID-19 vaccination during pregnancy, and concerns about safety were associated with hesitancy.[49–52] Based on the evidence of higher morbidity and mortality among pregnant persons with COVID-19, the American College of Obstetricians and Gynecologists and the Society for Maternal-Fetal Medicine issued guidance recommending both an initial vaccine series and booster vaccination for all eligible individuals regardless of pregnancy or lactation status.[53,54] Despite accumulating evidence of the safety and effectiveness of COVID-19 vaccination for pregnant persons and their offspring and the dangers of COVID-19 disease in pregnancy, as of June 18, 2022, the CDC estimated that 71% of pregnant people in the United States had received a COVID-19 vaccine, with 54.9% having received a booster dose and 3.1% having received at least one COVID-19 dose while pregnant.[55–57]

Children

In surveys done to date, parents are less accepting of COVID-19 vaccines for their children than for themselves. In general, surveys performed later in the pandemic in late 2021 showed greater levels of parental acceptance of COVID-19 vaccines compared with surveys performed in 2020 and early 2021.[29,58–67] A nationally representative survey of US parents in October-November 2021 found that for children ages 0 to 4 years, 52% of parents were likely to have their children vaccinated, and for ages 5% to 11% and 12% to 17%, 54% and 70% of parents, respectively, reported they were likely to vaccinate or had already vaccinated their children.[30] However, roughly 40% of parents with children 0 to 11 year old wanted to "wait and see" before vaccination, and another 36% would not let their children get a COVID-19 vaccine. Parents in that study who had received a COVID-19 vaccine themselves were 1.9, 3.7, and 6.2 times more likely to accept COVID-19 vaccination for their 0 to 4, 5 to 11, and 12- to 17-year-old children, respectively; however, this effect was not statistically significant for parents of children 0 to 4 years old, the age group for which a vaccine had not yet been authorized at the time of the study.[30] Acceptance of COVID-19 vaccination for children is also associated with acceptance of routine childhood immunizations and prior receipt of a seasonal influenza vaccine.[30]

Male parents, older parents, and parents of older children have higher rates of COVID-19 vaccine acceptance compared with female parents, younger parents, and parents of younger children.[59,68–70] Parents in the United States of Hispanic ethnicity are more likely to accept COVID-19 vaccination for children compared with non-Hispanic parents.[68,69,71,72] Compared with the United States, Canadian parents' acceptance of pediatric COVID-19 vaccines was initially higher, but that gap has narrowed with time.[31,73]

Parents must balance the perceived risks of COVID-19 disease against perceived risks and benefits of COVID-19 vaccination. The media often report that pediatric COVID-19 disease is mild, but parental perception that pediatric COVID-19 disease is severe is a predictor of positive vaccination intention for children 0 to 4 and 5 to 11.[30] At the same time, parents report concerns about the side effects of COVID-19 vaccines, and parents with attitudinal barriers to COVID-19 vaccination are less likely to accept the vaccine for their children.[29,30,62,67]

REASONS FOR CORONAVIRUS DISEASE-2019 VACCINE HESITANCY
Novelty of Vaccines

Several aspects of COVID-19 vaccination are distinct from other vaccines. First, SARS-CoV-2 is a novel human pathogen, and no vaccines for human coronaviruses had ever reached late-stage development in the past. Second, the mRNA and viral-vectored technologies applied to COVID-19 vaccines had been in development for decades preceding the emergence of SARS-CoV-2 but had not been used in vaccines previously authorized for the general population. Third, the process through which the biomedical research community moved from pathogen identification to successful vaccine development and production was not only unprecedented in terms of speed but also in terms of public visibility. Perceptions that the vaccines were "rushed," that the technologies were "too new," and that SARS-CoV-2 might "burn out" on its own or provide sustained natural immunity fed reluctance toward COVID-19 vaccines and have prompted a "wait and see" approach for many people who are otherwise not reluctant toward other vaccines.[74,75]

Safety Concerns

The high visibility of COVID-19 vaccination campaigns in the media amplified awareness of rare side effects following vaccination, beginning with anaphylaxis following mRNA vaccination.[76] The identification of serious blood clots, caused by the entity now known as vaccine-induced immune thrombotic thrombocytopenia, and Guillain-Barré syndrome in recipients of viral-vectored vaccines and of myopericarditis in adolescent and young adult males following mRNA vaccination created further concerns about vaccine safety.[77–82]

In addition to concerns about rare but immediate or proximate side effects, some reluctance stemmed from concern about unknown long-term side effects. Among these are concerns about effects on fertility spurred by rumors associating COVID-19 vaccines with both female and male infertility that became widespread on social media. Some were rooted in the rhetoric of past anti-vaccine campaigns about human papillomavirus (HPV) vaccines, whereas others capitalized upon fears of forced sterilizations among the Black American community.[83] Still others seized upon the rapidly expanding body of knowledge about SARS-CoV-2, drawing parallels between the spike protein and placental proteins and positing that vaccine-induced antibodies targeting the spike protein might also attack the placenta.[84] Studies have shown no adverse effects on either female or male fertility after COVID-19 vaccination, but public concerns persist.[50,83,85,86]

Beliefs about Susceptibility, Severity, and Effectiveness

From the first days of the COVID-19 pandemic, it was well known that the disease tended to be more severe in older populations, particularly when compared with children, and for a time, there was some evidence that children were less likely to become infected.[87] Thus, public perception that COVID-19 was a relatively benign illness in children was common and has contributed to parental resistance to vaccination.[30,31,61] In addition, as the COVID-19 vaccination campaign progressed and discussion of booster doses became public, some construed the need for boosters to mean that the vaccines were not effective. Contributing to this misperception in children specifically were the effectiveness results from the clinical trials in children, particularly those less than 5 years of age (or 6 for the Moderna vaccine).[88] When mRNA vaccines were eventually authorized for children less than age 5, the studies in this age group were done during the omicron wave, when vaccine effectiveness against infection was known to be relatively low compared with the initial studies in adults undertaken during circulation of the ancestral variant, which showed very high effectiveness against all outcomes, including infection.[89]

Religious and Philosophic Concerns

Although some groups argue against COVID-19 vaccine mandates on the grounds of personal liberty, others with reluctance around available COVID-19 vaccines have cited religious concerns about the vaccines.[90] Although essentially all major organized religions encourage vaccination with the available COVID-19 vaccines, groups with staunch objections to the use of embryonic stem cells in vaccine development and/ or manufacturing have voiced preferences for vaccines other than the mRNA and viral-vectored vaccines currently available in the United States.[91]

Misinformation and Disinformation Campaigns

Some false beliefs about COVID-19 disease and vaccines that contribute to hesitancy may result from the purposeful dissemination of disinformation; others stem from an abundance of readily available misinformation and may be informed by individual or group tendencies toward conspiratorial beliefs.[92] Some countries have denied the presence of COVID-19 within their borders altogether for the majority of the pandemic, but even in countries with high rates of COVID-19 transmission such as the United States, there are portions of the public that do not perceive COVID-19 to be a threat.[93,94] This may be due to local transmission dynamics, personal experiences of mild COVID-19 disease, or skepticism about the severity of COVID-19 disease among other possible reasons.[24,74,75] Conspiratorial beliefs about the contents and functions of the vaccines also weigh into the considerations of the risks of COVID-19 disease versus the risks of COVID-19 vaccines. Some of these include the idea that the vaccines might alter the recipient's DNA or allow a government or corporate entity to manipulate, control, or track the vaccine through the use of microchips.[24,74,75]

Politics and Trust

Breakdown of trust in authorities. Although social cohesion was initially galvanized by the perception of a common threat in the form of COVID-19, policy decisions in response to the pandemic became highly politicized and polarizing. In the United States and elsewhere, affiliation with right-leaning political parties has been associated with resistance to masking and COVID-19 vaccination, whereas left-leaning political parties largely promoted both interventions.[95,96] Political party affiliation may be used as a surrogate category to represent sociopolitical beliefs, but characterizing attitudes along party lines fails to account for large segments of the population that do not align with political parties, leaving gaps in our understanding of the ideological drivers of acceptance vs. reluctance toward COVID-19 vaccination.

A general breakdown in trust of authorities worldwide has not spared government officials and public health authorities responding to the pandemic. Roughly 40% of Americans in an April 2020 poll felt that both the CDC and the FDA paid too much attention to politics. Although in April 2020 83% of respondents to the same poll reported that they considered CDC to be a trustworthy source of reliable information about the coronavirus, 2 years later only 64% of those polled reported the CDC is a trustworthy source of reliable information on COVID-19 vaccines.[24,92]

Continued trust in personal health care providers. Despite a breakdown of trust in government and public health authorities, individual health care providers still garner high levels of confidence. A November 2021 poll found that 77% of US parents trusted their children's health care provider or pediatrician "a great deal" or "fair amount" to provide reliable information about COVID-19 vaccines for children, including 59% of unvaccinated parents.[29] The percentage of parents reporting trust in their children's pediatricians increased to 83% in April 2022%, and 85% of all US adults in the same poll reported trust in their own health care provider.[66]

Interventions to Improve Coronavirus Disease-2019 Vaccine Acceptance

Given the novelty of both the pathogen and the vaccines used to combat it, one challenge in addressing COVID-19 vaccine hesitancy is that the research and public health communities have had limited time to understand what works to improve confidence and uptake. We can apply best practices from other vaccines, such as strengthening patient-provider communication and community engagement campaigns, but more time and investigation are needed to determine whether some strategies work better than others. Framing communications around efficacy, side effects, and relative risks have been shown to influence COVID-19 vaccination preferences and acceptance among adults in general and may help encourage acceptance among parents deciding when and whether to vaccinate their children.[97,98] Behavioral nudges in the form of text message reminders improved adult COVID-19 vaccine uptake in two randomized controlled trials, although these interventions were targeting populations prioritized for vaccination, and the outcome was short-term uptake.[99] Similar recall-reminder strategies and the use of presumptive announcements have been shown to improve adherence to other recommended vaccines, including among pediatric populations.[100,101]

Surveys of parental acceptance show that parents who receive a recommendation from their children's health care provider are more likely to accept COVID-19 vaccination and that parents prefer for their younger children to receive a COVID-19 vaccine at their pediatric provider's office as opposed to a pharmacy, where the bulk of COVID-19 vaccines are currently delivered.[29,30,102] Although 85% of pediatricians are enrolled in the Vaccines for Children (VFC) program and two-third of VFC providers are enrolled to give COVID-19 vaccines, only 1/3 are actually delivering the vaccines.[102,103] Ensuring that young children have access to COVID-19 vaccines requires that pediatric providers not only have the capacity to stock the vaccines but also that they are actively recommending vaccination to their patients' families. Even among pediatric providers who do not stock the vaccine, their communication, advocacy, and assistance in getting children vaccinated is critical.

There are issues unique to COVID-19 vaccination of children relative to other childhood vaccines that may require novel interventions to improve uptake. There is a need to develop interventions to address concerns about novelty in a rapidly developed pandemic vaccine that would be relevant to both this and other pandemics. There are also specific issues unique to COVID-19 vaccination. For example, it is now well-known that myocarditis is associated with mRNA vaccines,[104,105] particularly for adolescent and young adult males. Although it is clear that the benefits of vaccination clearly outweigh this rare risk (ie, the risk of myocarditis from infection is much higher than from vaccination),[106] the risk is real, and many adolescents and young adults have been hospitalized as a result, a fact that has not been missed in both traditional and online media. Although other childhood vaccines can be associated with rare adverse events requiring hospitalization, these are very rare and not typically front-page news. Developing and testing interventions that can address these types of rare adverse events both during and outside of a pandemic is an important area for future research.

SUMMARY

Acceptance of every vaccine that is authorized, licensed, and recommended may be influenced by factors common to all vaccines and by factors unique to, or amplified by, the individual vaccine and the time during which it was developed and rolled out. COVID-19 vaccines were developed, manufactured, tested, authorized, distributed, and first administered amidst recurring waves of the pandemic. Some of the factors related to COVID-19 vaccine acceptance or reluctance that has been exaggerated relative to general vaccine acceptance or reluctance include the use of newer manufacturing technologies, politicization of many aspects of pandemic control, and the intense public and media scrutiny of every aspect of COVID-19 vaccine research and implementation. Future work on vaccine hesitancy should focus not only on the factors common to all vaccines, but also on factors that are unique or intensified in relation to vaccines directed against pathogens causing epidemics and pandemics.

CLINICS CARE POINTS

- Pediatricians should strongly recommend and offer coronavirus disease-2019 (COVID-19) vaccination.
- Do not assume that parents who accept routine childhood vaccines and/or COVID-19 vaccination for themselves will also accept COVID-19 vaccination for their children.
- When counseling parents on COVID-19 vaccination, it is important to understand (1) their perceptions about the risk of COVID-19 disease in themselves and their children and (2) their concerns about the risks of vaccination.

DISCLOSURE

Each individual listed as an author has contributed to the article to a significant extent in line with ICMJE guidelines. Dr. Hammershaimb drafted the outline with input from Drs. Campbell and O'Leary; Dr. Hammershaimb wrote the draft manuscript with input from Drs. Campbell and O'Leary. Dr. O'Leary revised the article based on the editor feedback. The submitted article was reviewed, edited, and agreed upon by all three authors.

FUNDING AND COMMERCIAL AND FINANCIAL INTERESTS

All authors will provide this information via a formal disclosure form, as noted in the instructions.

REFERENCES

1. World Health Organization. Novel Coronavirus (2019-nCoV) Situation Report - 1. 2020.
2. Dong E, Du H, Gardner L. An interactive web-based dashboard to track COVID-19 in real time. Lancet Infect Dis 2020;20(5):533–4.
3. Burki TK. The Russian vaccine for COVID-19. Lancet Respir Med 2020;8(11): e85–6.
4. Ledford H, Cyranoski D, Van Noorden R. The UK has approved a COVID vaccine - here's what scientists now want to know. Nature 2020;588(7837):205–6.
5. FDA Takes Key Action in Fight Against COVID-19 By Issuing Emergency Use Authorization for First COVID-19 Vaccine [press release]. December 11, 2020 2020.
6. China gives its first COVID-19 vaccine approval to Sinopharm. 2020.
7. Randolph HE, Barreiro LB. Herd Immunity: Understanding COVID-19. Immunity 2020;52(5):737–41.
8. Lazarus JV, Ratzan SC, Palayew A, et al. A global survey of potential acceptance of a COVID-19 vaccine. Nat Med 2020;27(2):354.
9. Hamel LKA, Muñana C, Brodie M. KFF COVID-19 vaccine monitor. Kaiser Family Foundation 2020;2020.

10. Dooling K, McClung N, Chamberland M, et al. The Advisory Committee on Immunization Practices' Interim Recommendation for Allocating Initial Supplies of COVID-19 Vaccine - United States, 2020. MMWR Morb Mortal Wkly Rep 2020; 69(49):1857–9.
11. Gharpure R, Guo A, Bishnoi CK, et al. Early COVID-19 First-Dose Vaccination Coverage Among Residents and Staff Members of Skilled Nursing Facilities Participating in the Pharmacy Partnership for Long-Term Care Program - United States, December 2020-January 2021. MMWR Morb Mortal Wkly Rep 2021; 70(5):178–82.
12. Lee JT, Althomsons SP, Wu H, et al. Disparities in COVID-19 Vaccination Coverage Among Health Care Personnel Working in Long-Term Care Facilities, by Job Category, National Health care Safety Network - United States, March 2021. MMWR Morb Mortal Wkly Rep 2021;70(30):1036–9.
13. Dzieciolowska S, Hamel D, Gadio S, et al. Covid-19 vaccine acceptance, hesitancy, and refusal among Canadian health care workers: A multicenter survey. Am J Infect Control 2021;49(9):1152–7.
14. Khubchandani J, Bustos E, Chowdhury S, et al. COVID-19 vaccine refusal among nurses worldwide: review of trends and predictors. Vaccines (Basel) 2022;10(2):230.
15. Biswas N, Mustapha T, Khubchandani J, et al. The nature and extent of covid-19 vaccination hesitancy in health care workers. J Community Health 2021;46(6): 1244–51.
16. Ciardi F, Menon V, Jensen JL, et al. Knowledge, attitudes and perceptions of covid-19 vaccination among health care workers of an inner-city hospital in new york. Vaccines (Basel) 2021;9(5):516.
17. Farah W, Breeher L, Shah V, et al. Disparities in COVID-19 vaccine uptake among health care workers. Vaccine 2022;40(19):2749–54.
18. Ashley Kirzinger AK, Liz Hamel, Mollyann Brodie. KFF/The Washington post frontline health care workers survey. 2021.
19. Caiazzo V, Witkoski Stimpfel A. Vaccine hesitancy in American health care workers during the COVID-19 vaccine roll out: an integrative review. Public Health 2022;207:94–104.
20. Warren AM, Perrin PB, Elliott TR, et al. Reasons for COVID-19 vaccine hesitancy in individuals with chronic health conditions. Health Sci Rep 2022;5(2):e485.
21. Aberumand B, Ayoub Goulstone W, Betschel S. Understanding attitudes and obstacles to vaccination against COVID-19 in patients with primary immunodeficiency. Allergy Asthma Clin Immunol 2022;18(1):38.
22. Nguyen KH, Srivastav A, Razzaghi H, et al. COVID-19 Vaccination Intent, Perceptions, and Reasons for Not Vaccinating Among Groups Prioritized for Early Vaccination - United States, September and December 2020. MMWR Morb Mortal Wkly Rep 2021;70(6):217–22.
23. Hamel LSA, Stokes M, Brodie M. KFF COVID-19 Vaccine Monitor: Vaccine Attitudes Among Essential Workers 2021;23:2021.
24. COVID-19 Vaccine Monitor Dashboard. Kaiser Family Foundation. Available at: https://www.kff.org/coronavirus-covid-19/dashboard/kff-covid-19-vaccine-monitor-dashboard/. Accessed Oct. 28, 2021.
25. Canada Go. Vaccine uptake in Canadian adults: Highlights from the 2020-2021 Seasonal Influenza Vaccination Coverage Survey. 2021.
26. New York Times. Available at: https://www.nytimes.com/interactive/2020/us/covid-19-vaccine-doses.html. Accessed July 29, 2022.

27. Centers of Disease Control and Prevention. Trends in Demographic Character-istics of People Receiving COVID-19 Vaccinations in the United States. Available at: https://covid.cdc.gov/covid-data-tracker/#vaccination-demographics-trends. Updated May 31, 2022. Accessed May 31, 2022.
28. Centers of Disease Control and Prevention. Pediatric Data. COVID Data Tracker Web site. 2021. Available at: https://covid.cdc.gov/covid-data-tracker/#pediatric-data. Accessed Oct. 28, 2021.
29. Liz Hamel LL, Kirzinger Ashley, Kearney Audrey, et al. KFF COVID-19 vaccine monitor: winter 2021 update on parents' views of vaccines for kids. Kaiser Fam Found 2021;9.
30. Hammershaimb EA, Cole LD, Liang Y, et al. COVID-19 Vaccine Acceptance Among US Parents: A Nationally Representative Survey. J Pediatr Infect Dis Soc 2022;11(8):361–70.
31. Humble RM, Sell H, Dube E, et al. Canadian parents' perceptions of COVID-19 vaccination and intention to vaccinate their children: Results from a cross-sectional national survey. Vaccine 2021;39(52):7669–76.
32. COVID-19 vaccination in Canada. Available at: https://health-infobase.canada.ca/covid-19/vaccination-coverage/. Accessed May 27, 2022.
33. Coronavirus (COVID-19) Update: FDA Authorizes Moderna and Pfizer-BioNTech COVID-19 Vaccines for Children Down to 6 Months of Age [press release]. June 17, 2022.
34. Delgado-Gallegos JL, Padilla-Rivas GR, Gastelum-Arias LJ, et al. Parent's Perspective towards Child COVID-19 Vaccination: An Online Cross-Sectional Study in Mexico. Int J Environ Res Public Health 2021;19(1):290.
35. Lopez O. As other nations push to vaccinate children, Mexico is an outlier. New York Times 2021.
36. Sargent RH, Laurie S, Moncada L, et al. Masks, money, and mandates: A national survey on efforts to increase COVID-19 vaccination intentions in the United States. PLoS One 2022;17(4):e0267154.
37. Pereira I. COVID-19 vaccine mandates moving the needle, experts say. In: ABC News.
38. Press JFaA. How Tyson Foods' CEO convinced 96% of his 120,000 employees to get vaccinated for COVID in just 3 months. Fortune; 2021.
39. Centers of Disease Control and Prevention. Risk for COVID-19 Infection, Hospitalization, and Death By Race/Ethnicity. 2021. Available at: https://www.cdc.gov/coronavirus/2019-ncov/covid-data/investigations-discovery/hospitalization-death-by-race-ethnicity.html. Accessed Mar. 15, 2021.
40. Prevention" CfDCa. Demographic Trends of COVID-19 cases and deaths in the US reported to CDC. 2021. Available at: https://covid.cdc.gov/covid-data-tracker/#demographics. Accessed October 28, 2021.
41. Bogart LM, Ojikutu BO, Tyagi K, et al. COVID-19 Related Medical Mistrust, Health Impacts, and Potential Vaccine Hesitancy Among Black Americans Living With HIV. J Acquir Immune Defic Syndr 2021;86(2):200–7.
42. Palamenghi L, Barello S, Boccia S, et al. Mistrust in biomedical research and vaccine hesitancy: the forefront challenge in the battle against COVID-19 in Italy. Eur J Epidemiol 2020;35(8):785–8.
43. Brandt AM. Racism and research: the case of the Tuskegee Syphilis Study. Hastings Cent Rep 1978;8(6):21–9.
44. Strodel R, Dayton L, Garrison-Desany HM, et al. COVID-19 vaccine prioritization of incarcerated people relative to other vulnerable groups: An analysis of state plans. PLoS One 2021;16(6):e0253208.

45. Testa A, Fahmy C. COVID-19 Mitigation Compliance and Vaccination Status Among Formerly Incarcerated Individuals in the United States. Health Educ Behav 2022;49(2):210–8.
46. Stern MF, Piasecki AM, Strick LB, et al. Willingness to Receive a COVID-19 Vaccination Among Incarcerated or Detained Persons in Correctional and Detention Facilities - Four States, September-December 2020. MMWR Morb Mortal Wkly Rep 2021;70(13):473–7.
47. Ortiz-Paredes D, Varsaneux O, Worthington J, et al. Reasons for COVID-19 vaccine refusal among people incarcerated in Canadian federal prisons. PLoS One 2022;17(3):e0264145.
48. COVID-19 vaccinations for prison populations and staff: Report on global scan. Penal Reform International and Harm Reduction International. 2021. Available at: https://www.europris.org/wp-content/uploads/2021/12/HRI-PRI_CovidVaccinationReport_Dec2021.pdf. Accessed July 29, 2022.
49. Cui Y, Binger K, Palatnik A. Attitudes and Beliefs Associated With COVID-19 Vaccination During Pregnancy. JAMA Netw Open 2022;5(4):e227430.
50. Kharbanda EO, Vazquez-Benitez G. COVID-19 mRNA Vaccines During Pregnancy: New Evidence to Help Address Vaccine Hesitancy. JAMA 2022;327(15):1451–3.
51. Reifferscheid L, Marfo E, Assi A, et al. COVID-19 vaccine uptake and intention during pregnancy in Canada. Can J Public Health 2022;113(4):547–58.
52. Gutierrez S, Logan R, Marshall C, et al. Predictors of COVID-19 Vaccination Likelihood Among Reproductive-Aged Women in the United States. Public Health Rep 2022;137(3):588–96.
53. ACOG and SMFM recommend COVID-19 vaccination for pregnant individuals [press release]. July 30, 2021.
54. ACoOa Gynecologists. COVID-19 Vaccination Considerations for Obstetric–Gynecologic Care. 2022. Available at: https://www.acog.org/clinical/clinical-guidance/practice-advisory/articles/2020/12/covid-19-vaccination-considerations-for-obstetric-gynecologic-care. Accessed May 31, 2022.
55. Goldshtein I, Steinberg DM, Kuint J, et al. Association of BNT162b2 COVID-19 Vaccination During Pregnancy With Neonatal and Early Infant Outcomes. JAMA Pediatr 2022;176(5):470–7.
56. Centers of Disease Control and Prevention. COVID-19 vaccination among pregnant people aged 18-49 years overall, by race/ethnicity, and date reported to CDC - Vaccine Safety Datalink, United States. 2022. Available at: https://covid.cdc.gov/covid-data-tracker/#vaccinations-pregnant-women. Accessed May 31, 2022.
57. Fu W, Sivajohan B, McClymont E, et al. Systematic review of the safety, immunogenicity, and effectiveness of COVID-19 vaccines in pregnant and lactating individuals and their infants. Int J Gynaecol Obstet 2022;156(3):406–17.
58. Goldman RD, Krupik D, Ali S, et al. Caregiver Willingness to Vaccinate Their Children against COVID-19 after Adult Vaccine Approval. Int J Environ Res Public Health 2021;18(19).
59. Rane MS, Robertson MM, Westmoreland DA, et al. Intention to Vaccinate Children Against COVID-19 Among Vaccinated and Unvaccinated US Parents. JAMA Pediatr 2022;176(2):201–3.
60. Chen F, He Y, Shi Y. Parents' and Guardians' Willingness to Vaccinate Their Children against COVID-19: A Systematic Review and Meta-Analysis. Vaccines (Basel) 2022;10(2).

61. Szilagyi PG, Shah MD, Delgado JR, et al. Parents' Intentions and Perceptions About COVID-19 Vaccination for Their Children: Results From a National Survey. Pediatrics 2021;148(4).
62. Ruggiero KM, Wong J, Sweeney CF, et al. Parents' Intentions to Vaccinate Their Children Against COVID-19. J Pediatr Health Care 2021;35(5):509–17.
63. Teasdale CA, Borrell LN, Kimball S, et al. Plans to Vaccinate Children for Coronavirus Disease 2019: A Survey of United States Parents. J Pediatr 2021;237: 292–7.
64. Teherani M, Banskota S, Camacho-Gonzalez A, et al. Intent to Vaccinate SARS-CoV-2 Infected Children in US Households. A Surv Vaccin (Basel) 2021;9(9).
65. Hamel L. LL, Sparks G., Stokes M., et al KFF COVID-19 Vaccine Monitor - April 2021. May 6, 2021 2021.
66. Sparks GMA, Lopes L, Hamel L, et al. KFF COVID-19 Vaccine Monitor - April 2022 2022;4:2022.
67. Liz Hamel LL, Grace Sparks, Kirzinger Ashley, et al. KFF COVID-19 Vaccine Monitor: 2021. Kaiser Fam Found 2021;28.
68. Kreuter MW, Garg R, Marsh A, et al. Intention to vaccinate children for COVID-19: A segmentation analysis among Medicaid parents in Florida. Prev Med 2022;156:106959.
69. Gray A, Fisher CB. Determinants of COVID-19 Vaccine Uptake in Adolescents 12-17 Years Old: Examining Pediatric Vaccine Hesitancy Among Racially Diverse Parents in the United States. Front Public Health 2022;10:844310.
70. Goldman RD, Ceballo R, International C-PASG. Parental gender differences in attitudes and willingness to vaccinate against COVID-19. J Paediatr Child Health 2022;58(6):1016–21.
71. McKinnon B, Quach C, Dube E, et al. Social inequalities in COVID-19 vaccine acceptance and uptake for children and adolescents in Montreal, Canada. Vaccine 2021;39(49):7140–5.
72. Fisher CB, Gray A, Sheck I. COVID-19 Pediatric Vaccine Hesitancy among Racially Diverse Parents in the United States. Vaccines (Basel) 2021;10(1).
73. Goldman RD, Bone JN, Gelernter R, et al. National COVID-19 vaccine program progress and parents' willingness to vaccinate their children. Hum Vaccin Immunother 2021;17(12):4889–95.
74. Tang L, Douglas S, Laila A. Among sheeples and antivaxxers: Social media responses to COVID-19 vaccine news posted by Canadian news organizations, and recommendations to counter vaccine hesitancy. Can Commun Dis Rep 2021;47(12):524–33.
75. CfDCa Prevention. Myths and Facts about COVID-19 Vaccines. 2022. Available at: https://www.cdc.gov/coronavirus/2019-ncov/vaccines/facts.html. Accessed June 24, 2022.
76. Shimabukuro TT, Cole M, Su JR. Reports of Anaphylaxis After Receipt of mRNA COVID-19 Vaccines in the US-December 14, 2020-January 18, 2021. JAMA 2021;325(11):1101–2.
77. T S. Thrombosis with thrombocytopenia syndrome (TTS) following Janssen COVID-19 vaccine. In. Advisory committee on immunization Practices. 2021.
78. American Society of Hematology. Vaccine-induced Immune Thrombotic Thrombocytopenia. 2022. Available at: https://www.hematology.org/covid-19/vaccine-induced-immune-thrombotic-thrombocytopenia. Updated May 9, 2022. Accessed.

79. Keh RYS, Scanlon S, Datta-Nemdharry P, et al. COVID-19 vaccination and Guillain-Barre syndrome: analyses using the National Immunoglobulin Database. Brain 2022;awac067.
80. Hanson KE, Goddard K, Lewis N, et al. Incidence of Guillain-Barre Syndrome After COVID-19 Vaccination in the Vaccine Safety Datalink. JAMA Netw Open 2022;5(4):e228879.
81. Oster ME, Shay DK, Su JR, et al. Myocarditis Cases Reported After mRNA-Based COVID-19 Vaccination in the US From December 2020 to August 2021. JAMA 2022;327(4):331–40.
82. Ontario PH. Myocarditis and Pericarditis after COVID-19 mRNA Vaccines. In:2022:1-17
83. Abbasi J. Widespread Misinformation About Infertility Continues to Create COVID-19 Vaccine Hesitancy. JAMA 2022;327(11):1013–5.
84. Head of Pfizer Research: Covid Vaccine is Female Sterilization. Health and Money News. 2020. Available at: https://healthandmoneynews.wordpress.com/2020/12/02/head-of-pfizer-research-covid-vaccine-is-female-sterilization/?fbclid=IwAR2HXbuZbKTR08HWnEV1wusabYR0d1ipKZF2ToaS71ScO7ugq8Z8gZDCIRk. Accessed May 31, 2022.
85. Lu-Culligan A, Tabachnikova A, Perez-Then E, et al. No evidence of fetal defects or anti-syncytin-1 antibody induction following COVID-19 mRNA vaccination. Plos Biol 2022;20(5):e3001506.
86. Safrai M, Herzberg S, Imbar T, et al. The BNT162b2 mRNA Covid-19 vaccine does not impair sperm parameters. Reprod Biomed Online 2022;44(4):685–8.
87. Davies NG, Klepac P, Liu Y, et al. Age-dependent effects in the transmission and control of COVID-19 epidemics. Nat Med 2020;26(8):1205–11.
88. Coronavirus (COVID-19) Update. FDA Authorizes Moderna and Pfizer-BioNTech COVID-19 Vaccines for Children Down to 6 Months of Age [press release]. Food Drug Adm 2022;17.
89. FDA Takes Key Action in Fight Against COVID-19 By Issuing Emergency Use Authorization for First COVID-19 Vaccine [press release]. Food Drug Adm 2020;11.
90. Religious Identities and the Race Against the Virus: American Attitudes on Vaccination Mandates and Religious Exemptions. Public Religion Res Inst Interfaith Youth Core 2021;9.
91. J J. New Novavax Shot Could Appeal to Pro-Life Christian Skeptics. In. Christianity Today.
92. Liz Hamel AK, Kirzinger Ashley, Lopes Lunna, et al. KFF Health Tracking Poll - September 2020: Top Issues in 2020 Election, The Role of Misinformation, and Views on A Potential Coronavirus Vaccine. Kaiser Fam Found 2020;10.
93. Hashim HT, El Rassoul AEA, Bchara J, et al. COVID-19 denial in Turkmenistan veiling the real situation. Arch Public Health 2022;80(1):8.
94. Smith A. Kim Jong Un says pandemic has caused 'great crisis' in North Korea. NBC News 2021;30.
95. Stoler J, Klofstad CA, Enders AM, et al. Sociopolitical and psychological correlates of COVID-19 vaccine hesitancy in the United States during summer 2021. Soc Sci Med 2022;306:115112.
96. Albrecht D. Vaccination, politics and COVID-19 impacts. BMC Public Health 2022;22(1):96.
97. Kreps S, Kriner DL. Communication about vaccine efficacy and COVID-19 vaccine choice: Evidence from a survey experiment in the United States. PLoS One 2022;17(3):e0265011.

98. Thorpe A, Fagerlin A, Drews FA, et al. Communications to Promote Interest and Confidence in COVID-19 Vaccines. Am J Health Promot 2022;36(6):976–86.
99. Dai H, Saccardo S, Han MA, et al. Behavioural nudges increase COVID-19 vaccinations. Nature 2021;597(7876):404–9.
100. Szilagyi PG, Thomas K, Shah MD, et al. National Trends in the US Public's Likelihood of Getting a COVID-19 Vaccine-April 1 to December 8, 2020. JAMA 2020; 325(4):396–8.
101. Brewer NT, Hall ME, Malo TL, et al. Announcements Versus Conversations to Improve HPV Vaccination Coverage: A Randomized Trial. Pediatrics 2017; 139(1):e20161764.
102. Oliver S. Updates to the Evidence to Recommendation Framework: Pfizer-BioNTech COVID-19 booster in children aged 5-11 years. In. Advisory committee on immunization practices: Centers for Disease Control and Prevention.
103. O'Leary S.T., Allison M.A., Vogt T., et al., Pediatricians' experiences with and perceptions of the vaccines for children program, *Pediatrics*, 145 (3), 2020, e20191207.
104. Mevorach D, Anis E, Cedar N, et al. Myocarditis after BNT162b2 mRNA Vaccine against Covid-19 in Israel. N Engl J Med 2021;385(23):2140–9.
105. Mevorach D, Anis E, Cedar N, et al. Myocarditis after BNT162b2 Vaccination in Israeli Adolescents. N Engl J Med 2022;386(10):998–9.
106. Patone M, Mei XW, Handunnetthi L, et al. Risks of myocarditis, pericarditis, and cardiac arrhythmias associated with COVID-19 vaccination or SARS-CoV-2 infection. Nat Med 2022;28(2):410–22.

Vaccine Hesitancy in Specific Groups

Maternal Vaccination and Vaccine Hesitancy

Cynthia M. Rand, MD, MPH[a],*, Courtney Olson-Chen, MD, MS[b]

KEYWORDS

- Prenatal care • Vaccination • Vaccination hesitancy • Tdap vaccine
- Influenza vaccine • COVID-19 vaccine

KEY POINTS

- Influenza, Tdap, and COVID-19 vaccines are safe to give during pregnancy.
- These vaccines provide protection to newborns via transplacental transfer and prevent maternal morbidity caused by influenza and COVID-19.
- Obstetric care providers should stock vaccine in their office to increase vaccination rates.
- Obstetric care providers and their office staff should continue to offer vaccines even if a pregnant person refused the vaccine previously.
- Vaccine safety is the most common concern for patients; future studies in vaccine communication and counseling for obstetric care providers are needed.

INTRODUCTION

Vaccination is an essential part of the care of pregnant patients. No adverse fetal impacts have been identified with inactivated virus, toxoid, or bacterial vaccines. Live-attenuated vaccines should be reserved for the postpartum period.[1] The American College of Obstetrics and Gynecology (ACOG) recommends that both inactivated influenza vaccine and Tdap are given during every pregnancy and that all pregnant individuals are vaccinated against COVID-19. Specifically, the influenza vaccine is recommended during each influenza vaccination season as soon as it becomes available. It can be given in any trimester. The ideal window to receive Tdap extends from 27 to 36 weeks gestation to maximize passive antibody transfer for the newborn.[1] COVID vaccine, including boosters, is recommended any time during pregnancy when a patient is eligible. The most recent US estimates of pregnancy vaccination rates, from 2019 to 2020, showed 61.2% of pregnant people received the influenza vaccine, 56.6% received Tdap, and 40.3% received both vaccines.[2] COVID-19 rates of full vaccination among pregnant people were last reported to be above 70%, with the

[a] Department of Pediatrics, University of Rochester Medical Center, 601 Elmwood Avenue, Box 777, Rochester, NY 14642, USA; [b] Department of Obstetrics & Gynecology, University of Rochester Medical Center, 601 Elmwood Avenue, Box 668, Rochester, NY 14642, USA
* Corresponding author.
E-mail address: cynthia_rand@urmc.rochester.edu

Pediatr Clin N Am 70 (2023) 259–269
https://doi.org/10.1016/j.pcl.2022.11.004
0031-3955/23/© 2022 Elsevier Inc. All rights reserved.
pediatric.theclinics.com

majority of people now fully vaccinated before pregnancy.[3] Significant racial disparities in full vaccination coverage for COVID remain, with 89.5% of Asians being fully
vaccinated before or during pregnancy, 67.9% among White, and 58.1% among
Black pregnant people.[3]

For influenza and Tdap vaccine, the highest vaccination rates were among those who
received a provider offer or referral for vaccination. Racial and ethnic disparities in pregnancy vaccination rates are particularly notable for the Tdap vaccine with 35.8%
coverage among Hispanic women and 38.8% among Black women compared with
65.5% of White women. Data from the Pregnancy Risk Assessment Monitoring Systems
survey showed that after adjustment for factors including maternal age, marital status,
education, prenatal care utilization, and smoking, Black women were 30% less likely to
receive the influenza vaccine compared with non-Hispanic White women.[4] In addition,
women living in rural areas were less likely to receive influenza vaccination during pregnancy.[5] Overall, approximately 40% of pregnant people do not receive influenza and
Tdap vaccines, which leaves them vulnerable to maternal and neonatal infection. An
analysis of National Health Interview Survey (NHIS) data from 2012 to 2018 showed
that the strongest predictor of vaccination during pregnancy was having health insurance, followed by having a higher income and greater level of education.[6]

DISCUSSION
Influenza

Pregnancy increases the risk of morbidity and mortality related to influenza infection; it
is associated with physiologic changes including decreased lung capacity and
increased cardiac output that leave patients vulnerable to the impacts of influenza
infection.[7] This was particularly notable during the H1N1 pandemic when pregnant
people were more likely to be hospitalized and also more likely to die from the infection
compared with those who were not pregnant.[8]

Large cohorts of pregnant patients have been followed after inactivated influenza
vaccination. There is no association between vaccination and adverse pregnancy outcomes including cesarean delivery, preterm birth, or infant medical conditions up to
6 months of age.[9] Longitudinal prospective studies of influenza vaccination in pregnancy following children up to 7 years of age found no increase in congenital malfor-
mations, malignancies, or neurocognitive delays.[7]

Prior studies have shown that inactivated influenza vaccine is effective in reducing
hospitalization in pregnancy by an average of 40%.[10] Not only does the vaccine prevent maternal infection but also transplacental influenza antibody transfer occurs and
provides protection for newborns who cannot receive the vaccine before 6 months of
age.[7,8] A recent meta-analysis showed that maternal influenza vaccination was associated with an overall reduction of influenza infection in infants of 34%.[11] In addition,
administration of the influenza vaccine during pregnancy is associated with a
deceased risk of preterm birth and low birth weight infants.[12]

Despite the value of vaccination, pregnant people have low influenza vaccination
rates. Health care workers effect the decisions of patients when they are considering
influenza vaccination. They can play an important role in protecting pregnant people
and their infants from a vaccine-preventable disease. Understanding and communicating the safety and efficacy of influenza vaccine is essential.[7]

Tdap

The ACOG recommends that all pregnant patients receive a Tdap vaccine during each
pregnancy to prevent pertussis in infants[1] as the infant pertussis vaccination series

does not begin until 2 months of age. When Tdap vaccine is given as early as possible in the 27 to 36 weeks of gestation window, it benefits the neonate by passive transfer of antibodies across the placenta.[1]

A large retrospective cohort found that the maternal Tdap vaccination was highly protective against pertussis infection in infants, particularly in the first 2 months of life.[13] There was 91.4% effectiveness among infants during the first 2 months and 69% during the first year of life. The protection from hospitalization was 94% and from pertussis-related death was 95%. Providing Tdap immunization during pregnancy is even more effective for protecting newborns compared with "cocooning," in which people with close contact to the infant are vaccinated (eg, postpartum maternal vaccination) as a form of infant protection.[13]

A systematic review of 1.4 million pregnant patients who received the Tdap vaccine investigated its safety. Those receiving the vaccine had no increased risk for adverse birth outcomes, including preterm birth. The study found a slightly higher incidence of chorioamnionitis in those who received Tdap; fever following the vaccine was reported in up to 3% of pregnant patients.[14] Risk ratios for chorioamnionitis were small and did not seem to be clinically relevant. A more recent retrospective review of 5 years of birth data in Ontario, Canada, found no association with chorioamnionitis or other adverse events.[15]

COVID-19

Following the release of the initial COVID-19 vaccines in December 2020, multiple national and international societies representing obstetric and reproductive health care providers released a unified statement supporting public health measures to combat COVID-19, which included the emergency authorized use of COVID-19 vaccines in pregnancy. The group also urged the inclusion of pregnant people in vaccine trials.[16] In July 2021, the centers for disease control and prevention (CDC) released new data on the safety of COVID-19 vaccination in pregnancy, and at this time, the ACOG officially announced a strong recommendation for the COVID-19 vaccine in pregnancy.[17]

A systematic review of mRNA COVID-19 vaccines given during pregnancy included more than 48,000 subjects and demonstrated that both the Pfizer-BioNTech and Moderna vaccines can prevent SARS-CoV-2 infection in pregnant people.[18] The most common adverse reactions were similar to the general population and included pain at the injection site, fatigue, and headache. In a systematic review, pregnant people who received COVID-19 vaccine during pregnancy did not have a higher risk of adverse pregnancy or neonatal outcomes compared with unvaccinated pregnant people.[19]

In addition to effectiveness in prevention of maternal COVID-19 during pregnancy, the vaccine has been associated with a decrease in the stillbirth rate.[20] In a systematic review, antibody responses were rapid after the first vaccine dose. After the second dose, antibody responses were stronger and associated with better transplacental antibody transfer. Longer intervals between first vaccination dose and delivery were also associated with higher antibody fetal IgG measured in cord blood and a better antibody transfer ratio.[18] Maternal completion of the two-dose COVID-19 vaccination series during pregnancy was associated with a decrease in hospitalization among infants less than 6 months of age.[21] In addition, vaccinations conferred protective immunity to newborns through breast milk.[19] COVID-19 vaccination in pregnancy has clearly demonstrated both maternal and neonatal benefit, though future studies are needed to clarify optimal timing as well as utility of repeat vaccination during pregnancy.

Vaccination Disparities and Reasons for Hesitancy

Numerous factors contribute to lower uptake of influenza vaccine among Black nonpregnant adults that carry over into vaccine hesitancy during pregnancy; the key factors include attitudes and beliefs, knowledge, lack of access, trust in health care providers and vaccines, risk perception, and racial discrimination.[22] Historical medical injustices and ongoing racial discrimination contribute to mistrust of the health care system.[23] For pregnant people, research has shown that compared with White women, Black and Hispanic women were less confident in vaccine safety and efficacy and less likely to trust information from health care providers and public health authorities.[24] Black women were the least confident in the safety of the maternal influenza and Tdap vaccine. This is important, as women with higher confidence in vaccine safety and efficacy for themselves and their infant, as well as those with higher perceived risk of influenza and pertussis disease had greater intention to receive flu and Tdap vaccines (four to nine times greater odds of vaccine acceptance).[25,26] In addition, those pregnant for the first time were less sure of their vaccine knowledge and intentions than those with prior children. In a meta-analysis of factors that influence maternal vaccination in pregnancy believing there was potential for vaccine-induced harm had a negative influence on seasonal influenza vaccine uptake (OR 0.22, 95% CI 0.11–0.44) and reduced the odds of being vaccinated fivefold.[25] Prior influenza vaccination is a strong predictor of influenza vaccination during pregnancy[27]; the odds of receiving an influenza vaccine during pregnancy are three to five times greater if an individual receives an influenza vaccine outside of pregnancy. Factors specifically associated with increased Tdap vaccination include receiving an influenza vaccination, having the vaccine available on-site at the obstetrician's office, and having a higher number of prenatal care visits.[28,29]

A health care provider recommendation is one of the strongest predictors of immunization during pregnancy for both influenza and Tdap.[28,30] A meta-analysis of factors that influence vaccine decision-making for pregnant women found the odds of receiving a pertussis or influenza vaccination are 10 to 12 times higher among pregnant women who received a provider recommendation.[25] Black women historically report a lower rate of being recommended or offered influenza vaccine during pregnancy,[31] and among those offered, Black women are less likely to receive the vaccine compared with other women.[2] In addition, receipt of a provider offer or referral for Tdap during pregnancy was lower among Black than among Hispanic women and White women in 2020. Among those with a provider offer for Tdap vaccination, coverage was lowest for Hispanic women, followed by Black women, and White women.[2]

Influenza Vaccine Hesitancy

In a 2016 survey of obstetric providers, the most commonly reported reasons for vaccine refusal were patients' belief that influenza vaccine makes them sick (48%), belief they are unlikely to get a vaccine-preventable disease (38%), general worries about vaccines (32%), desire to maintain a natural pregnancy (31%), and concern that their child could develop autism as a result of vaccination during pregnancy (25%).[32] The extrapolation of autism fears to vaccination in pregnancy highlights the potential impact of vaccine safety misinformation. Many obstetric providers believed that stressing the potential harm of disease to the newborn was most effective in conversations with patients. The patient concerns reported by providers match those that have been reported directly by patients.[33] Specifically, patients worry about side effects for themselves and potential harm for their fetus; some have concerns about vaccine ingredients, such as mercury, and some believe the vaccine is not effective at preventing influenza disease.[34]

COVID Vaccine Hesitancy Reasons

Because pregnant people were not included in COVID-19 vaccine clinical trials, the advice regarding receipt of COVID vaccine for pregnant people changed rapidly over the course of 2020 to 21. During the early years of the pandemic, pregnant patients who were Black, Hispanic, younger, with lower education, prior refusal of the influenza vaccine, or who were not counseled about the COVID vaccination had lower vaccine acceptance.[19,35]

Studies have examined reasons for COVID vaccine hesitancy during pregnancy, some of which are the same as those for nonpregnant patients, and some of which are specific to pregnancy. Most commonly, women who are hesitant report lack of information about vaccine safety during pregnancy,[35] on fetal development, and on later child well-being.[36] Conversely, the predictors of vaccine acceptance include confidence in vaccine safety and effectiveness, worrying about COVID-19, compliance to mask guidelines, trust of public health agencies, and positive attitudes toward routine vaccines.[37]

Specific Issues Related to Pregnancy

Specific issues related to pregnancy care offer opportunities to increase vaccination rates. For most patients, office visits during pregnancy are frequent, with 12 to 14 visits recommended during a healthy pregnancy. Visits tend to be monthly during the first 4 to 28 weeks, then every other week from 28 to 36 weeks gestation, and weekly thereafter. During the COVID-19 pandemic, a shift toward telemedicine visits occurred to limit exposure to the virus; some offices recommended 6 or fewer in-person visits during pregnancy, with alternate visits offered virtually.[38,39] The first prenatal visit is longer and more comprehensive, allowing an opportunity to discuss healthy living and health care, including vaccinations, during pregnancy.[40] The influenza vaccine is often offered at the first prenatal visit is seasonally appropriate, and some offices combine the 28-week glucose test for diabetes with an opportunity to give the Tdap vaccine. If patients refuse either the influenza or Tdap vaccine, vaccination can be discussed again at future visits as patients are seen frequently.

Increasing evidence shows that many parents make decisions about vaccines for their children during pregnancy, or even before conception.[41–43] One study of low-income pregnant women found that half considered pregnancy to be the best time to receive information about childhood vaccination and were most likely to indicate the nurse who gave them vaccines as the person with whom they would like to discuss childhood vaccines.[44] More research is needed to assess the feasibility of having discussions of childhood vaccines in the obstetric office as well as the willingness of obstetric nurses and providers to take on this role.

Evidence to Overcome Vaccine Hesitancy/Increase Rates

Several approaches aimed at increasing maternal vaccination rates during pregnancy have been successful (**Table 1**). As noted above, a provider recommendation is the most important predictor of vaccine uptake for pregnant people.[45] However, there is a gap in communication training for obstetric providers, with little or no training available in how best to communicate with vaccine-hesitant patients.[46] Regarding specific communication techniques, studies show that message framing (loss- or gain-framed) in isolation is not an effective intervention.[47,48] In a survey of obstetricians, the most commonly reported strategies used to address refusal were stating that it is safe to receive vaccines in pregnancy (96%), explaining that not getting the vaccine puts the fetus or newborn at risk (90%) or not getting the vaccine puts the pregnant

Table 1 Evidence for interventions to increase maternal vaccination rates	
Intervention	**Evidence**
Provider recommendation	++
Stocking vaccines in practice	++
Standing orders	+
Group prenatal care	+
Offering vaccination more than once	+
Provider prompt	+
Multifaceted QI intervention	+
Patient education	+/−
Patient reminders	+/−

Strong evidence (++); Some evidence (+); No evidence (−).

person's health at risk (84%).[32] The strategy perceived as most effective was stating that not getting vaccinated puts the fetus or newborn at risk. In addition, it is necessary to continue to offer vaccine despite refusal; in one study, 20% of pregnant people who received influenza vaccine had previously refused it.[49] Emphasizing the need for vaccination more than once helps patients realize its importance.

In a systematic review that examined interventions to increase influenza vaccination rates, educational interventions aimed at pregnant people resulted in higher rates in half of studies.[50] Many interventions have been tried, including pamphlets, text messages, video, and apps for pregnant individuals.[48,51–54] Two studies using educational pamphlets increased vaccination rates; the pamphlets discussed flu vaccine safety and the benefit of the vaccine to the pregnant person and the infant.[51,55] Educational text messaging[56] and video-based education[54] did not improve rates. It remains unclear how best to educate pregnant individuals to increase vaccine uptake and how to combat misinformation.

Several studies of mothers have found that information focusing on the benefit and safety of vaccines given to pregnant people to protect their infant is beneficial and preferred to information about protecting the pregnant person.[55,57] A different approach is to target-specific concerns; an app-based intervention that provided videos based on parent needs was well received by pregnant people, even among those who were vaccine hesitant; this has not yet been shown to increase vaccination rates.[58] Patients use CDC and pregnancy Websites for vaccine information, but they value information from their providers.[59]

Other practice-based interventions that can be effective include changing the model of care to group visits, offering reminders to patients, prompting providers, and having standing orders in place. Stocking vaccines in the practice is also associated with increased uptake,[60] so patients do not have to make separate appointments or travel to off-site locations for vaccination. A study of group prenatal care found a much higher rate of influenza vaccine uptake (62% vs 38%) in the group model compared with traditional care group.[61] The increase was attributed to both more patient education and social support.

Reminders for pregnant patients to return for vaccines have been shown to be effective in one study. Specifically, text message reminders in the fall increased influenza vaccination uptake during pregnancy.[53] In a public health campaign, Text4Baby, computerized reminders that pregnant people sign up for online, increased influenza vaccination during pregnancy, particularly for those whose provider had not recommended the vaccine.[62] Such reminders can serve as a way to message patients who have fewer health care visits.

Office-based interventions have the potential to increase vaccination rates. In one study, a prompt to the provider from the electronic health record was associated with a dramatic increase in Tdap vaccination at 32 weeks gestation; this occurred at a time when recommendations changed from offering the vaccine from postnatal to prenatal, so the prompt was not tested alone.[63] In addition, standing orders have been shown to be effective for both Tdap and influenza vaccine.[64,65] Given that many electronic health record (EHRs) have checklists to indicate specific tests done during pregnancy, using such a list or other easily visible documentation has the potential to serve as a reminder to staff and providers as well.

More than one approach is likely necessary to dramatically increase rates, as is needed for childhood and adolescent vaccines.[66] One example of combining multiple interventions is the AFIX-OB intervention.[67] This program was modeled after the CDCs AFIX QI program. It provided QI strategies (eg, standing order, EHR reminder), technical assistance with immunization champions, incentives, and practice-based tools. The program was successful in increasing rates of influenza and Tdap vaccination rates in two states. It is important to see if such interventions can be scaled-up to affect a larger population in a cost-effective way.

SUMMARY

Vaccination during pregnancy is critical for both maternal and neonatal protection as many vaccines cannot be administered until 2 to 6 months after birth. Although pregnant patients were excluded from many initial vaccination safety studies, growing safety data are reassuring for inactivated influenza, Tdap, and COVID-19 vaccination. There are known racial disparities in vaccination rates, with Black women often having lower rates compared with women of other races; efforts must be made to make health care during pregnancy equitable. Vaccine hesitancy has many potential sources, but effective strategies to overcome hesitancy include directed obstetric provider recommendations, improved access, and continuing to offer vaccine. Additional research is needed specifically focused on communication with vaccine-hesitant pregnant patients.

CLINICS CARE POINTS

- Personal vaccination recommendations from obstetric providers are crucial.
- Vaccination discussions that focus on the safety and benefit for the infant are preferred by pregnant individuals.
- Providers should offer vaccines even if previously refused as patients may be more accepting later in pregnancy.
- Stocking vaccine in the obstetric provider office is needed to increase rates.
- Standing orders can be used as an effective way to increase vaccination rates.
- A multipronged approach that includes effective communication as well as workflow changes is likely needed to increase vaccination rates for pregnant individuals.

DISCLOSURE

The authors have no conflicts of interest to disclose.

REFERENCES

1. ACOG committee opinion No. 741: maternal immunization. Obstet Gynecol 2018; 131(6):e214–7.
2. Razzaghi H, Kahn KE, Black CL, et al. Influenza and tdap vaccination coverage among pregnant women - United States, April 2020. MMWR Morb Mortal Wkly Rep 2020;69(39):1391–7.
3. COVID-19 vaccination among pregnant people aged 18-49 years overall, by race/ethnicity, and date reported to CDC- vaccine safety datalink, United States. CDC; 2022. Available at: https://covid.cdc.gov/covid-data-tracker/#vaccinations-pregnant-women. [Accessed 8 June 2022]. Accessed.
4. Arnold LD, Luong L, Rebmann T, et al. Racial disparities in U.S. maternal influenza vaccine uptake: results from analysis of pregnancy risk assessment monitoring system (PRAMS) data, 2012-2015. Vaccine 2019;37(18):2520–6.
5. Kaur R, Callaghan T, Regan AK. Disparities in maternal influenza immunization among women in rural and urban areas of the United States. Prev Med 2021; 147:106531.
6. Cambou MC, Copeland TP, Nielsen-Saines K, et al. Insurance status predicts self-reported influenza vaccine coverage among pregnant women in the United States: a cross-sectional analysis of the National Health Interview Study Data from 2012 to 2018. Vaccine 2021;39(15):2068–73.
7. Tamma PD, Ault KA, del Rio C, et al. Safety of influenza vaccination during pregnancy. Am J Obstet Gynecol 2009;201(6):547–52.
8. Jamieson DJ, Honein MA, Rasmussen SA, et al. H1N1 2009 influenza virus infection during pregnancy in the USA. Lancet 2009;374(9688):451–8.
9. Munoz FM, Greisinger AJ, Wehmanen OA, et al. Safety of influenza vaccination during pregnancy. Am J Obstet Gynecol 2005;192(4):1098–106.
10. Thompson MG, Kwong JC, Regan AK, et al. Influenza vaccine effectiveness in preventing influenza-associated hospitalizations during pregnancy: a multi-country retrospective test negative design study, 2010-2016. Clin Infect Dis 2019;68(9):1444–53.
11. Jarvis JR, Dorey RB, Warricker FDM, et al. The effectiveness of influenza vaccination in pregnancy in relation to child health outcomes: systematic review and meta-analysis. Vaccine 2020;38(7):1601–13.
12. Nunes MC, Aqil AR, Omer SB, et al. The effects of influenza vaccination during pregnancy on birth outcomes: a systematic review and meta-analysis. Am J Perinatol 2016;33(11):1104–14.
13. Baxter R, Bartlett J, Fireman B, et al. Effectiveness of vaccination during pregnancy to prevent infant pertussis. Pediatrics 2017;139(5):e20164091.
14. Vygen-Bonnet S, Hellenbrand W, Garbe E, et al. Safety and effectiveness of acellular pertussis vaccination during pregnancy: a systematic review. BMC Infect Dis 2020;20(1):136.
15. Fakhraei R, Crowcroft N, Bolotin S, et al. Obstetric and perinatal health outcomes after pertussis vaccination during pregnancy in Ontario, Canada: a retrospective cohort study. CMAJ Open 2021;9(2):E349.
16. American Association of Gynecologic Laparoscopists. AAGL joint statement supporting public health measures to combat COVID-19. Cypress, CA: American Association of Gynecologic Laparoscopists; 2020. Available at: https://www.aagl. org/press-releases-statements/joint-statement-supporting-public-health-measures-to-combat-covid-19/. Accessed June 8, 2022.

17. American College of Obstetricians and Gynecologists. ACOG COVID_19 vaccines and pregnancy: conversation guide. Washington, DC: ACOG; 2021. Available at: https://www.acog.org/covid-19/covid-19-vaccines-and-pregnancy-conversation-guide-for-clinicians. Accessed June 9, 2022.
18. Pratama NR, Wafa IA, Budi DS, et al. mRNA Covid-19 vaccines in pregnancy: a systematic review. PLoS One 2022;17(2):e0261350.
19. Rawal S, Tackett RL, Stone RH, et al. COVID-19 vaccination among pregnant people in the United States: a systematic review. Am J Obstet Gynecol MFM 2022;4(4):100616.
20. Prasad S, Kalafat E, Blakeway H, et al. Systematic review and meta-analysis of the effectiveness and perinatal outcomes of COVID-19 vaccination in pregnancy. Nat Commun 2022;13(1):2414.
21. Halasa NB, Olson SM, Staat MA, et al. Effectiveness of maternal vaccination with mRNA COVID-19 vaccine during pregnancy against COVID-19-Associated hospitalization in infants aged <6 Months - 17 states, july 2021-january 2022. MMWR Morb Mortal Wkly Rep 2022;71(7):264–70.
22. Quinn SC, Jamison A, An J, et al. Breaking down the monolith: understanding flu vaccine uptake among African Americans. SSM Popul Health 2018;4:25–36.
23. Armstrong K, Putt M, Halbert CH, et al. Prior experiences of racial discrimination and racial differences in health care system distrust. Med Care 2013;51(2): 144–50.
24. Dudley MZ, Limaye RJ, Salmon DA, et al. Racial/ethnic disparities in maternal vaccine knowledge, attitudes, and intentions. Public Health Rep 2021;136(6): 699–709.
25. Kilich E, Dada S, Francis MR, et al. Factors that influence vaccination decision-making among pregnant women: a systematic review and meta-analysis. PLoS One 2020;15(7):e0234827.
26. Dudley MZ, Limaye RJ, Omer SB, et al. Characterizing the vaccine knowledge, attitudes, beliefs, and intentions of pregnant women in Georgia and Colorado. Hum Vaccin Immunother 2020;16(5):1109–17.
27. Bartolo S, Deliege E, Mancel O, et al. Determinants of influenza vaccination uptake in pregnancy: a large single-centre cohort study. BMC Pregnancy Childbirth 2019;19(1):510.
28. Wales DP, Khan S, Suresh D, et al. Factors associated with Tdap vaccination receipt during pregnancy: a cross-sectional study. Public Health 2020;179: 38–44.
29. Ghaswalla P, Poirrier JE, Packnett ER, et al. Maternal immunization in the U.S.: a nationwide retrospective cohort study. Am J Prev Med 2019;57(3):e87–93.
30. Henninger ML, Irving SA, Thompson M, et al. Factors associated with seasonal influenza vaccination in pregnant women. J Womens Health (Larchmt) 2015; 24(5):394–402.
31. Callahan AG, Coleman-Cowger VH, Schulkin J, et al. Racial disparities in influenza immunization during pregnancy in the United States: a narrative review of the evidence for disparities and potential interventions. Vaccine 2021;39(35): 4938–48.
32. O'Leary ST, Riley LE, Lindley MC, et al. Obstetrician-gynecologists' strategies to address vaccine refusal among pregnant women. Obstet Gynecol 2019; 133(1):40–7.
33. Chamberlain AT, Seib K, Ault KA, et al. Factors associated with intention to receive influenza and tetanus, diphtheria, and acellular pertussis (Tdap) vaccines during pregnancy: a focus on vaccine hesitancy and perceptions of disease

severity and vaccine safety. PLoS Curr 2015;7. https://doi.org/10.1371/currents.outbreaks.d37b61bceebae5a7a06d40a301cfa819.

34. Lutz CS, Carr W, Cohn A, et al. Understanding barriers and predictors of maternal immunization: identifying gaps through an exploratory literature review. Vaccine 2018;36(49):7445–55.

35. Battarbee AN, Stockwell MS, Varner M, et al. Attitudes toward COVID-19 illness and COVID-19 vaccination among pregnant women: a cross-sectional multi-center study during august-december 2020. Am J Perinatol 2022;39(1):75–83.

36. Simmons LA, Whipps MDM, Phipps JE, et al. Understanding COVID-19 vaccine uptake during pregnancy: 'hesitance', knowledge, and evidence-based decision-making. Vaccine 2022;40(19):2755–60.

37. Skjefte M, Ngirbabul M, Akeju O, et al. COVID-19 vaccine acceptance among pregnant women and mothers of young children: results of a survey in 16 countries. Eur J Epidemiol 2021;36(2):197–211.

38. Fryer K, Delgado A, Foti T, et al. Implementation of obstetric telehealth during COVID-19 and beyond. Matern Child Health J 2020;24(9):1104–10.

39. Peahl AF, Zahn CM, Turrentine M, et al. The michigan plan for appropriate tailored healthcare in pregnancy prenatal care recommendations. Obstet Gynecol 2021;138(4):593–602.

40. American Academy of Pediatrics ACoOaG. Guidelines for perinatal care. 8th edition. Elk Grove Village (IL): American Academy of Pediatrics; The American College of Obstetricians and Gynecologists; 2017.

41. Yarnall JN, Seashore C, Phillipi CA, et al. Timing of vaccine decision-making among first-time parents. Acad Pediatr 2022;22(4):551–8.

42. Corben P, Leask J. Vaccination hesitancy in the antenatal period: a cross-sectional survey. BMC Public Health 2018;18(1):566.

43. Rubincam C, Greyson D, Haselden C, et al. Is the pre-natal period a missed opportunity for communicating with parents about immunizations? Evidence from a longitudinal qualitative study in Victoria, British Columbia. BMC Public Health 2022;22(1):237.

44. Fuchs EL, Hirth JM, Guo F, et al. Infant vaccination education preferences among low-income pregnant women. Hum Vaccin Immunother 2021;17(1):255–8.

45. Chamberlain AT, Seib K, Ault KA, et al. Improving influenza and Tdap vaccination during pregnancy: a cluster-randomized trial of a multi-component antenatal vaccine promotion package in late influenza season. Vaccine 2015;33(30):3571–9.

46. Frawley JE, McKenzie K, Sinclair L, et al. Midwives' knowledge, attitudes and confidence in discussing maternal and childhood immunisation with parents: A national study. Vaccine 2020;38(2):366–71.

47. Frew PM, Saint-Victor DS, Owens LE, et al. Socioecological and message framing factors influencing maternal influenza immunization among minority women. Vaccine 2014;32(15):1736–44.

48. Frew PM, Kriss JL, Chamberlain AT, et al. A randomized trial of maternal influenza immunization decision-making: A test of persuasive messaging models. Hum Vaccin Immunother 2016;12(8):1989–96.

49. Goggins ER, Williams R, Kim TG, et al. Assessing influenza vaccination behaviors among medically underserved obstetric patients. J Womens Health (Larchmt) 2021;30(1):52–60.

50. Ellingson MK, Dudley MZ, Limaye RJ, et al. Enhancing uptake of influenza maternal vaccine. Expert Rev Vaccin 2019;18(2):191–204.

51. Meharry PM, Cusson RM, Stiller R, et al. Maternal influenza vaccination: evaluation of a patient-centered pamphlet designed to increase uptake in pregnancy. Matern child Health J 2014;18(5):1205–14.
52. Moniz MH, Hasley S, Meyn LA, et al. Improving influenza vaccination rates in pregnancy through text messaging: a randomized controlled trial. Obstet Gynecol 2013;121(4):734–40.
53. Stockwell MS, Westhoff C, Kharbanda EO, et al. Influenza vaccine text message reminders for urban, low-income pregnant women: a randomized controlled trial. Am J Public Health 2014;104(Suppl 1):e7–12.
54. Goodman K, Mossad SB, Taksler GB, et al. Impact of video education on influenza vaccination in pregnancy. J Reprod Med 2015;60(11–12):471–9.
55. Yudin MH, Salripour M, Sgro MD. Impact of patient education on knowledge of influenza and vaccine recommendations among pregnant women. J Obstet Gynaecol Can 2010;32(3):232–7.
56. Jordan ET, Bushar JA, Kendrick JS, et al. Encouraging influenza vaccination among text4baby pregnant women and mothers. Am J Prev Med 2015;49(4):563–72.
57. Fuss TL, Devera JL, Pierre-Joseph N, et al. Attitudes and communication preferences for vaccines among pregnant women receiving care at a safety-net hospital. Women's health issues 2022;32(1):67–73.
58. Salmon DA, Limaye RJ, Dudley MZ, et al. Momstalkshots: an individually tailored educational application for maternal and infant vaccines. Vaccine 2019;37(43):6478–85.
59. Ellingson M, Chamberlain AT. Beyond the verbal: pregnant women's preferences for receiving influenza and Tdap vaccine information from their obstetric care providers. Hum Vaccin Immunother 2018;14(3):767–71.
60. Ding H, Black CL, Ball S, et al. Influenza vaccination coverage among pregnant women - United States, 2016-17 influenza season. MMWR Morb Mortal Wkly Rep 2017;66(38):1016–22.
61. Roussos-Ross D, Prieto A, Goodin A, et al. Increased Tdap and influenza vaccination acquisition among patients participating in group prenatal care. J Prim Prev 2020;41(5):413–20.
62. Bushar JA, Kendrick JS, Ding H, et al. Text4baby influenza messaging and influenza vaccination among pregnant women. Am J Prev Med 2017;53(6):845–53.
63. Morgan JL, Baggari SR, Chung W, et al. Association of a best-practice alert and prenatal administration with tetanus toxoid, reduced diphtheria toxoid, and acellular pertussis vaccination rates. Obstet Gynecol 2015;126(2):333–7.
64. Ogburn T, Espey EL, Contreras V, et al. Impact of clinic interventions on the rate of influenza vaccination in pregnant women. J Reprod Med 2007;52(9):753–6.
65. Patel KM, Vazquez Guillamet L, Pischel L, et al. Strategies to increase uptake of maternal pertussis vaccination. Expert Rev Vaccin 2021;20(7):779–96.
66. Rand CM, Humiston SG. Provider focused interventions to improve child and adolescent vaccination rates. Acad Pediatr 2021;21(4S):S34–9.
67. Spina CI, Brewer SE, Ellingson MK, et al. Adapting center for disease control and prevention's immunization quality improvement program to improve maternal vaccination uptake in obstetrics. Vaccine 2020;38(50):7963–9.

A Structural Lens Approach to Vaccine Hesitancy and Identity

Jennifer D. Kusma, MD, MS[a],*, Leslie Walker-Harding, MD[b],
Maria Veronica Svetaz, MD, MPH[c,d],
Tamera Coyne-Beasley, MD, MPH[e]

KEYWORDS

- Vaccine hesitancy • Culture • Identity

KEY POINTS

- It is essential to understand identity-based considerations around vaccines to improve understanding and communication around vaccine hesitancy.
- Applying critical consciousness can help create awareness among clinicians and help expand understanding of where this "hesitancy" comes from to serve everyone better.
- Identity-based considerations toward vaccines include those from varying racial and ethnic experiences, religious backgrounds, and contemporary socio-politico constructs.
- Using an identity-based lens can inform conversations about vaccines and help improve dialog around access to vaccines for all individuals.

INTRODUCTION

Vaccine hesitancy is defined by the World Health Organization (WHO) as the questioning or refusal of vaccines.[1] In practice, this can range from questioning one vaccine to all recommended vaccines, and it was cited by the WHO as among the top 10 threats to global health.[2] In an attempt to define the breadth of vaccine hesitancy, the SAGE group defined the "three C model," which includes confidence, convenience, and complacency.[1] Looking into each of these, confidence applies to a general trust or

[a] Division of Advanced General Pediatrics and Primary Care, Department of Pediatrics, Ann & Robert H. Lurie Children's Hospital of Chicago and Northwestern University Feinberg School of Medicine, 225 East Chicago Avenue, Box 162, Chicago, IL 60611, USA; [b] Department of Pediatrics, Seattle Children's, 4800 Sand Point Way NE, RB.2.401, Seattle, WA 98105, USA; [c] Department of Family and Community Medicine, Hennepin Healthcare, 516 Delaware Street SE, Minneapolis, MN 55455, USA; [d] Department of Family and Community Medicine, University of Minnesota, 1600 7th Avenue South, CPP1 310, Birmingham, AL 35233, USA; [e] Division of Adolescent Medicine, Department of Pediatrics, University of Alabama at Birmingham, Birmingham, AL, USA
* Corresponding author.
E-mail address: jkusma@luriechildrens.org

Pediatr Clin N Am 70 (2023) 271–282
https://doi.org/10.1016/j.pcl.2022.11.005
0031-3955/23/© 2022 Elsevier Inc. All rights reserved.
pediatric.theclinics.com

mistrust in vaccines, convenience is the physical availability of and access to vaccines, and complacency deals in the perceived risk of vaccine preventable illness.[1] Research shows that cultural themes are also essential to consider when evaluating vaccine hesitancy.[3] These themes around culture stem from a need to address the origins of a general mistrust to all health care among communities and the fact that for many, their preferences and values have not been honored systematically by the health-care systems. Cultural issues do not stem from culture per se; they originate from traumatic experiences linked with prior and current structural racism and biases that have plagued our health-care systems. This team of authors recommends the addition of a fourth C: critical consciousness (CC), aiming to create awareness that clinicians need to expand their understanding of where this "hesitancy" comes from to serve everyone better. Thus, we are going to refer to them not as cultural themes but as identity-based considerations.

Based on their training and decision-making, social workers have already integrated CC into evidence-based interventions, to keep their commitment to social justice. Since the Institute of Medicine's "Unequal Treatment," health care has been wrestling with how to fix differential care and outcomes. The COVID-19 pandemic accelerated the need to move solutions faster, as the pandemic marked racial, ethnic, and geographical disparities, becoming a syndemic. In Social Work, CC has become central to clinical decision-making:

> ... Sakamoto and Pitner (2005) argue that the practice of critical consciousness challenges social workers to be aware of the power they have and how this power is experienced in relation to those served. Such active critical awareness and analysis of power differentials is purposeful in the social worker's efforts to support the power of those served. To that end, critical consciousness requires intentional and ongoing self-reflection that addresses one's perception of self and others, social location and identities, relational intersections, forces of oppression within the environment, bias, assumptions, and the dynamics of power and privilege.[4]

Nursing have done the same to their pedagogy.[5] By adding CC to the model, we propose applying a cultural, identity-based lens to the 3-C model to help address vaccine hesitancy, with principles that can be applied more broadly and equitably, as defined above. To do this, there is urgency in training children and adolescent health-care professionals in a framework that considers mistrust and misinformation beyond the original 3-C model and incorporating structural perspectives that address how identity-related values were missed in the care equation. This includes building on strengths of individuals and communities and engaging in practices that promote equity, resilience, and health.

There are distinct lived experiences of oppression and discrimination that correlate with different identities. Various resources (bias training, clinical tools such as the ADDRESSING tool, and so forth) ensure that clinicians are mindful of their identities, their patients' identities, and the "isms" related to them. These lived experiences are relevant and must be considered when thinking about the background and foundation of being vaccine hesitant or health-care hesitant, and they can be informed by historic and current bias, racism, cultural or religious beliefs, and community norms (ie, politicization or ableism). These considerations vary across and within different identities: racial, ethnic, religious, and socio-politico groups, as well as across different vaccines, routine versus seasonal, and available vaccine modalities. Application of a conceptual model that uses identity constructs of vaccine hesitancy can allow us to see where trust intercepts with vaccine questioning or acceptance.[6] Ultimately, by learning about the perspectives of others toward vaccines and health care in general, clinicians gain, by using their CC, a crucial understanding of where concerns are rooted. This, in turn, will allow clinicians and families to work together in a critically conscious, antiracist, culturally, and linguistically sensitive manner to address concerns. The goal of this article is to broadly review identity-based considerations toward immunizations in the United States as a starting point toward vaccine cultural awareness, including antioppressive and antiracist considerations. There is intersectionality with culture, experiences of racism and bias, and access to health care. Barriers and poor quality of services also affect vaccine access and vaccine hesitancy within the cultural groups discussed and must be remembered in initiatives to address vaccine hesitancy. Although it is not possible to cover every individual's unique perspective toward vaccines, we attempt to describe perspectives on vaccines from the points of view of different lived experiences: racial and ethnic perspectives, religious perspectives, and contemporary socio-political cultural topics to help understand cultural considerations.

Racial and Ethnic Lived Experiences Considerations

There are distinct cultural perspectives toward vaccines and health care for individuals of varying racial and ethnic backgrounds for many reasons including historical and lived exploitation and mistrust. Among many individuals, including but not limited to Black, Indigenous, and Latine[a] individuals, there is significant mistrust in the healthcare system that is justified and rooted in historical and contemporary inequities and institutional and societal racism.[7,8]

Among many Black families and individuals in the United States, there is well-founded mistrust in health-care and government programs.[3,9,10] Black exploitation in medicine, documented from the centuries of slavery in the United States and extending into the current era, include having numerous medical experiments and surgeries conducted on their bodies and tissue samples without their knowledge or consent. These exemplify reasons for mistrust based on lived and vicarious experiences.[11] It is understandable that there is considerable mistrust in government and health care, especially with respect to infectious diseases. Past experiences that have negatively influenced the trust in health care among the Black community can be illustrated by one more well-known exploitation, the Tuskegee syphilis trials in which individuals were not provided with standard of care treatment of syphilis from the 1930s to 1970s, resulting in unnecessary disease burden and suffering.[12] Black parents endorsed that knowledge of the Tuskegee trials, and other medical exploitation of Black individuals, contributes to fear that their own child might be being experimented on with vaccines.[13]

Research studies have asked Black individuals and their families, through focus groups and interviews, about their perspectives and experiences with vaccines. In one focus group study, families expressed concern that they do not get adequate information about vaccines.[14] In other studies, it has been highlighted that Black parents have concerns that their children get lower quality vaccines than their peers.[14,15] When asked about why they do choose to vaccinate their children, despite fears, Black families that endorsed feeling like vaccines are required by society or school had a higher likelihood of parental willingness to get vaccines despite their mistrust.[13] As such, in a national survey study, it was found that race and ethnicity were not significantly associated with hesitancy toward school

---

[a] Language matters, and although there is not an overall consensus on terms, after careful consideration, we opted for the term Latine because it is gender inclusive and gaining respect among Latine community organizations.

required routine childhood vaccines.[16] To that end, when looking at vaccine data from the Centers for Disease Control and Prevention for 13 to 17-year olds from 2015 to 2019, Black teenagers have higher rates of receiving at least one meningitis vaccine when compared with their White counterparts and had higher rates of human papilloma virus (HPV) vaccine series completion when compared with White teens,[17] although the effect of the COVID-19 pandemic on these vaccine rates is not yet known.

It should be noted that social determinants of health are intimately intertwined with racism in the United States. For this reason, both access to health care and the way it is delivered have been compromised.[18–20] Poor access to health care and inequitable school systems are examples of root causes of low vaccine uptake.

The Latine community is broad, with heritage in multiple continents and countries including the United States, Central America, South America, the Caribbean, and Spain. These were categorized together based on policy surrounding the US Census in the 1970s.[21] As such, when discussing the Latine cultural perspective toward vaccines, it is important to consider that there are both unique and common cultural concerns among the many distinct populations that make up this community.[22] Mistrust has been augmented by medical malfeasance, cruelty, and exploitation of the Latine community, for example, when, as part of medical experiments, individuals in Guatemala were purposefully infected with sexually transmitted infections through direct exposure and inoculation.[23]

Research in the United States has shown that among immigrant populations, there tends to be lower rates of vaccination.[24] There are unique issues across different immigrant populations, which often include concerns that face those who are undocumented living in the United States.[22] Regardless of country of origin, the Latine community in the United States has high rates of uninsured or underinsured, so access to health care is a clear barrier. Among some, there are concerns about anti-immigrant policy and immigrant detainees concerns.[25] Research has shown that individuals who speak English as a second language express desire to receive vaccine information in their own language.[26] Therefore, information in a needed language serves as a second access barrier. Similar to Black families, once Latine families are able to obtain access to health care, they often find that the workforce neither reflects the community racial and ethnic distribution nor is the workforce cultural responsive. Clinicians offering advice may use the wrong undesired targets for change among the population they are serving. For example, focusing on individualistic goals (eg, "You will live longer") may not be persuasive for people who value inclusive-family-centered goals or inspire change in communities with group identity.

Asian American and Pacific Islanders (AAPI) and American Indian/Alaskan Native (AI/AN) are 2 additional heterogenous populations, in which making broad assumptions about vaccine hesitancy or willingness can miss important cultural differences and distinctions. Specifically, often Native Hawaiians and Pacific Islanders are not considered independently but rather included together with all AAPI individuals. Native Hawaiian and Pacific Islanders have been found to have significant vaccine hesitancy, especially concerning the COVID-19 vaccine.[27] Distinctions in vaccine hesitancy are missed when all AAPI populations are considered together,[28] further emphasizing the importance of the individual, identity-based approach. There is a history of unethical research conducted among AI/AN, and as a result, tribes have had hesitancy toward medical research.[29] Additionally, when looking at vaccine trends according to the Indian Health Service National Immunization Program, routine childhood vaccine through 2 years old have been decreasing and currently are at less than 60%

coverage.[30] Understanding the heterogenous nature of these cultures is important when considering vaccine hesitancy.

Religious Views and Objections

The United States has many diverse religions and spiritual belief systems.[31] This is important to consider because religious exemptions are a common mechanism for avoidance of routine childhood vaccines while maintaining school enrollment despite vaccine requirements. Currently there are 44 states with religious exemptions, and 15 states with moral or philosophical exemptions.[32]

One example of religious considerations is concerns from observant Jewish, Muslim, and Seventh Day Adventist communities about vaccines that contain gelatin that may have porcine origins that would be in opposition to their faith observations and dietary laws.[33] Additional concerns were raised around the COVID-19 vaccine from the Somali community in Minnesota, a largely Muslim community, who was concerned that receiving the COVID-19 vaccine would be considered breaking their Ramadan fast in addition to concerns that the vaccine had porcine elements—both in discordance with their faith.[34] Among Jewish groups, specifically those who are Orthodox and live in Orthodox communities, there are concerns about observing kosher dietary practices if receiving porcine-containing vaccines. Orthodox Jewish and Muslim communities have seen outbreaks of vaccine preventable illnesses. There were large measles outbreaks in a largely Muslim-Somali community in Minnesota in 2017,[35] and in the large Orthodox Jewish population in Rockland County, New York in 2018.[36,37] In 2022, the Rockland County Orthodox Jewish community has seen cases of polio, a disease previously considered eradicated from the United States in 1994.[38]

An additional religious consideration that has been raised by some is the inclusion of fetal embryo fibroblasts in vaccines. The concerns are raised by Catholic and other Christian communities about the cell origin being from aborted fetuses. The fetal cells used in vaccine development originated decades ago and were used in 3 of the routine childhood vaccines used today (hepatitis A, rubella, varicella).[39] Today, there are misunderstandings that fetal cells are contained within the vaccines; however, the cells were used in the research for some vaccines and are not in vaccines administered to the public.

The Amish community in America is another distinct cultural-religious community with overall low vaccine rates. Within Amish communities in the United States, there are overall lower rates of vaccination, and higher rates of vaccine preventable illnesses. In 2014, there was a measles outbreak in an Amish community in Ohio, where it was estimated that only 14% of affected households had measles-mumps-rubella vaccination coverage with even a single dose.[40] In a survey of Amish Americans, although one-third cited religious reasons for vaccine hesitancy, the majority were concerned that there were too many side effects or vaccines had dangerous preservatives in them.[41] Other studies have found similar concerns from parents about the safety profile of vaccines being the reason for hesitancy rather than religious concerns.[42] Amish communities surveyed have endorsed that if there was access to immunizations within their community, they would be willing to receive them.

It is important to emphasize that knowing a family's religion does not imply what an individual family may believe and/or practice regarding vaccines any more than knowing their race and ethnicity. There are many variations within religious communities on vaccine acceptance and hesitancy. It is important to meet each patient with an approach that allows them to let the provider know if there are religious considerations in immunization with their children or adolescents.

Contemporary Socio-Politico Cultural Concerns

There have been shifting socio-politico cultural interests and concerns during the last decade that must also be considered regarding vaccine hesitancy. First, there has been a growing mistrust in the medical and pharmaceutical fields, and a growing interest in natural product and immunity. This translates into vaccine hesitancy and includes questioning the inclusion of thimerosal and its safety in vaccines.[43] Studies have shown the safety of inclusion of thimerosal in vaccines; however, it has been removed from most vaccines to help increase comfort with vaccines.[44] There are also questions of the inclusion of aluminum, other metals, and formaldehyde in small quantities in vaccines.[45–47]

There has also been politicization of vaccines and vaccine requirements, with substantial vaccine hesitancy now falling along US political party affiliations, especially regarding the COVID-19 vaccine.[48,49] In addition to growing political polarization, there is distrust of government and authoritarianism that have also contributed to vaccine hesitancy. Studies of uptake of the COVID-19 vaccine found that political identification and political leaning of news exposure affected the likelihood of vaccine hesitancy.[48,50] General mistrust in vaccines may also stem from the H1N1 swine flu in 1976, in which there was concern about whether the vaccine efforts were for political purposes rather than public health need.[51] Public commentary at that time described the vaccine effort as a "sorry debacle," over concerns about large investments in a quick vaccine effort, with a vaccine that resulted in some who received it becoming ill.[52]

With the advent of the Internet and quick access to information, there has been an increase in the spread of misinformation and disinformation online and on social media.[53] Among the misinformation readily available, there is mounting and significant concerns among parents about common side effects of vaccines, such as swelling, rash, crying, and pain,[13] and some parents endorsing concerns about serious side effects, all of which is readily visible on social media.[16] In some communities and online, concerns about rare side effects are perceived as more immediate or grave than the no longer often visible infections,[54] including unsubstantiated, untrue claims of effects on fertility.[55]

From a cultural perspective, there are unique concerns and challenges that face rural communities.[24] Access is a large barrier for rural communities; there tends to be fewer pediatric practices and practices may have more of a challenge covering the costs of vaccine storage and administration.[24] Within rural communities, it is also important to consider the unique challenges of migrant working communities, where consistent access may vary.[22]

Discussion and Next Steps

Cultural considerations are a key factor in whether a family is hesitant toward vaccines. Culture and sense of self-identity are paramount in making medical decisions for each individual and their family, and as such, understanding different beliefs among groups that make up the United States is critical to help answer questions regarding optimal vaccine acceptance and administration. We propose the following to help reach communities where they are regarding vaccine questioning.

First, health-care providers and community leaders must work together with individuals of diverse backgrounds to promote trust. One step toward doing this includes increasing enrollment of racially and ethnically diverse individuals in vaccine clinical trials and having more trials led by racially and ethnically diverse investigators. This ensures that everyone is represented, and it improves the visibility and acceptability of vaccines—individuals can see that the vaccine is safe *for them* and not just *for others*. Research has shown that Black survey respondents would be more comfortable about a vaccine if it had more testing on individuals of their own race and ethnicity.[56]

Next, we must ensure equitable access of vaccines into all communities. This includes the distribution and availability of vaccines in community locations and working on a process that ensures the vaccines are distributed to members of the community and include administration at a variety of sites in the community.

We must recognize the existence of medical misconduct in the United States and abroad and acknowledge that a community's shared history can lead them to mistrust of the government and the health-care system. As health-care providers, we can engage with members of the community that can then serve as trusted messengers on the safety and importance of vaccines.[8] It is important to include groups of under-represented providers, not typically represented in decision-making, in the medical community. Provider–patient cultural concordance leads to improved medical out-comes and increased confidence in the health-care system. For example, among Lat-ine women, they endorsed being more likely to receive the HPV vaccine if the provider recommending it was woman and Latine.[57] Having information available in the preferred language of patients and having cultural navigators can help decrease bar-riers to vaccines. The COVID-19 vaccine programs in AI/AN populations demonstrate the success of working together with tribal leaders to improve COVID-19 vaccine up-take, with high rates of COVID-19 vaccine uptake among this community.[58] COVID-19 vaccine success has been attributed to allowing tribes to manage their own vaccine roll out, allowing for tribal autonomy that could account for tribal heterogeneity.[59] Vaccination efforts also considered tribal cultural considerations including the signif-icance of elders and traditional healers.[59]

Vaccines must be readily available and accessible to all communities. We know that social determinants of health are exacerbated in the setting of systemic racism, and families facing social challenges may have a harder time accessing routine care.[19,60] Healthy People 2030 aims to address social determinants of health as a means of improving health equity,[18] and as such, it is important that vaccines are readily available and are accessible to families at all time points at which they interact with the health-care system, even outside of well child visits.

Work must also be done to partner with religious communities, another form of iden-tity. We can work together with religious leaders to codesign and address concerns from each religious community. Although many religious organizations have made statements in favor of their followers being vaccinated,[61–63] it is important to collabo-rate with local religious leaders to best share the same message so that this message reaches all followers. Having religious leaders engage in public speaking on the reli-gious support of vaccination, or public receipt of vaccines may help followers feel more comfortable with vaccines.

Another way to address concerns rooted in religious identity is offering vaccines at religious centers. This may help congregants understand the religious acceptance of vaccines. This may also lead to increased access to vaccines, for example, in the Amish community where it has been said that if vaccines were more readily available, there would be interest in receiving them.[42] Additionally, providers being culturally aware of the religious stance on vaccines of some of their patients and acknowledging it could improve provider–parent–patient relationships.

Providers must encourage questions and conversation during primary care encoun-ters and all visits where vaccines are discussed. Understanding patients' identity and their view on vaccines can help clinicians navigate conversations about the safety and importance of vaccination in a way that is culturally and linguistically sensitive. It is important to include all staff of the clinical site as vaccine champions in learning, messaging, and advocating on the importance of vaccines and the exploration of their patient's perception of them. This should include medical assistants, patient service representatives, and administrative staff. In doing so, we increase the chances of patients connecting with a member of the health-care team, feeling like their concerns are heard, and feeling more comfortable with receiving vaccines. There is evidence in health care that concordant providers (eg, same race, same ethnicity) available to families improve health outcomes. Members of the health-care team should also reflect the composition of the community served.

There is also significant work to do outside of the health-care setting and offices to promote vaccine equity and cultural humility. To get out the message regarding vaccines, and to share information about its safety and importance in the community we should promote parents and teens from these communities to be trained as vaccine experts and advocates. They can help communicate through social media and in person about vaccines and provide insights into the best setting and best messaging that will resonate within the community. Providers should be visible in the communities they serve. Engagement in the community—through listening, volunteering, interacting, or advocating—allows providers to be known entities within the community. This, in turn, helps them be a credible source of trusted information if vaccine hesitancy or an outbreak of a vaccine preventable illness arises.

In addition to engagement in communities, it is important to engage with political and media leaders to spread helpful information and combat misinformation that is circulating about vaccines. Additionally, providers can be a vital community resource and should find ways to volunteer to be a source of information in political and media settings. Having information available across platforms, from television to cellular phones, from news and other information vehicles to social media, and from public service announcements and information pages on the Internet, will help to get good, credible information in the places that people often turn to formulate their opinions.[64] By interacting with the community and media, providers can also provide reassurance, for example, about the safety of stabilizing products in vaccines such as aluminum.

The COVID-19 pandemic has exacerbated health inequities across the United States while also revealing high COVID-19 vaccine hesitancy specifically among populations most effected by the pandemic. Doctors have been found to be an important source of information about the COVID-19 vaccine, emphasizing the importance of having vaccine conversations with patients and families.[64,65]

SUMMARY

An overarching theme in looking at culture, identity, and vaccines is that it is important not to make assumptions about families or any individuals questioning vaccines. As providers, CC about the different perspectives on vaccines that are prominent in various communities can help guide conversations with patients and their families and communities. Understanding the mistrust and misinformation around vaccines gives providers an opportunity to have truthful conversations with patients on the benefits and importance of vaccines.

Providers must remain open, present, and nonjudgmental in their conversations with individuals about vaccines. Do not make assumptions about an individual's vaccine attitudes just based on their identification with a particular group. Conversations about vaccines should be critically conscious, culturally appropriate, participatory, equity-focused, and linguistically sensitive. It is imperative to collaborate with families and communities to create a stronger shared understanding of vaccines, their safety profiles, and importance in combating disease in children and adolescents.

FINANCIAL DISCLOSURE

None of the authors has any commercial or financial relationships relevant to this article to disclose.

REFERENCES

1. MacDonald NE, Hesitancy SWGoV. Vaccine hesitancy: Definition, scope and determinants. Vaccine 2015;33(34):4161–4. https://doi.org/10.1016/j.vaccine.2015.04.036.
2. World Health Organization (WHO). Ten threats to global health. 2019. Available at: https://www.who.int/news-room/spotlight/ten-threats-to-global-health-in-2019. Accessed November 24, 2020.
3. Quinn S, Jamison A, Musa D, et al. Exploring the continuum of vaccine hesitancy between african american and white adults: results of a qualitative study. PLoS Curr 2016;8. https://doi.org/10.1371/currents.outbreaks.3e4a5ea39d8620494e2a2c874a3c4201.
4. O'Neill M. Applying critical consciousness and evidence-based practice decision-making: a framework for clinical social work practice. J Social Work Educ 2015;51(4):624–37.
5. Blanchet Garneau A, Browne AJ, Varcoe C. Drawing on antiracist approaches toward a critical antidiscriminatory pedagogy for nursing. Nurs Inq 2018;25(1). https://doi.org/10.1111/nin.12211.
6. Dube E, Laberge C, Guay M, et al. Vaccine hesitancy: an overview. Hum Vaccin Immunother 2013;9(8):1763–73.
7. Santibanez TA, Nguyen KH, Greby SM, et al. Parental vaccine hesitancy and childhood influenza vaccination. Pediatrics 2020. https://doi.org/10.1542/peds.2020-007609.
8. Coyne-Beasley T, Hill SV, Zimet G, et al. COVID-19 Vaccination of adolescents and young adults of color: viewing acceptance and uptake with a health equity lens. J Adolesc Health 2021;68(5):844–6.
9. Jamison AM, Quinn SC, Freimuth VS. You don't trust a government vaccine": narratives of institutional trust and influenza vaccination among African American and white adults. Soc Sci Med 2019;221:87–94.
10. Lin C, Tu P, Terry TC. Moving the needle on racial disparity: COVID-19 vaccine trust and hesitancy. Vaccine 2022;40(1):5–8.
11. Washington HA. Medical apartheid : the dark history of medical experimentation on Black Americans from colonial times to the present. 1st pbk. New York: Harlem Moon; 2006. p. 501, x.
12. Centers for Disease Control and Prevention (CDC). The U.S. Public health service syphilis study at tuskegee. 2021. Available at: https://www.cdc.gov/tuskegee/index.html. Accessed August 17, 2022.
13. Shui I, Kennedy A, Wooten K, et al. Factors influencing African-American mothers' concerns about immunization safety: a summary of focus group findings. J Natl Med Assoc 2005;97(5):657–66.
14. Shui IM, Weintraub ES, Gust DA. Parents concerned about vaccine safety: differences in race/ethnicity and attitudes. Am J Prev Med 2006;31(3):244–51.

15. Katz IT, Bogart LM, Fu CM, et al. Barriers to HPV immunization among blacks and latinos: a qualitative analysis of caregivers, adolescents, and providers. BMC Public Health 2016;16(1):874.

16. Kempe A, Saville AW, Albertin C, et al. Parental hesitancy about routine childhood and influenza vaccinations: a national survey. Pediatrics 2020;146(1). https://doi. org/10.1542/peds.2019-3852.

17. Centers for Disease Control and Prevention (CDC). TeenVaxView: vaccination coverage among adolescents (13 - 17 Years). 2021. Available at: https://www. cdc.gov/vaccines/imz-managers/coverage/teenvaxview/data-reports/index.html. Accessed September 1, 2022.

18. Warren MD, Hirai AH, Lee V. Accelerating upstream together: achieving infant health equity in the United States by 2030. Pediatrics 2022;149(2). https://doi. org/10.1542/peds.2021-052800.

19. Adler NE, Glymour MM, Fielding J. Addressing social determinants of health and health inequalities. JAMA 2016;316(16):1641–2.

20. Trent M, Dooley DG, Douge J, Section On Adolescent H, Council On Community P, Committee On A. The impact of racism on child and adolescent health. Pediatrics 2019;144(2). https://doi.org/10.1542/peds.2019-1765.

21. Hugo Lopez M, Manuel Krogstad J, Passel JS. Who is Hispanic?. 2021. Available at:https://www.pewresearch.org/fact-tank/2021/09/23/who-is-hispanic/.   .   Accessed August 31, 2022..

22. Ortiz AC, Akgun KM, Bazan IS. Embracing the diversity of latinx communities to promote vaccinations. Yale J Biol Med 2022;95(2):257–63.

23. Rodriguez MA, Garcia R. First, do no harm: the US sexually transmitted disease experiments in Guatemala. Am J Public Health 2013;103(12):2122–6.

24. Albers AN, Thaker J, Newcomer SR. Barriers to and facilitators of early childhood immunization in rural areas of the United States: a systematic review of the literature. Prev Med Rep 2022;27:101804.

25. Sanchez G, Peña J. Skepticism and mistrust challenge COVID vaccine uptake for Latinos. 2021. Available at: https://www.brookings.edu/blog/how-we-rise/2021/01/25/skepticism-and-mistrust-challenge-covid-vaccine-uptake-for-latinos/.   Accessed August 17, 2022.

26. Greenfield LS, Page LC, Kay M, et al. Strategies for increasing adolescent immunizations in diverse ethnic communities. J Adolesc Health 2015;56(5 Suppl): S47–53.

27. Samoa RA, Ethoan LN, Saw A, et al. Socioeconomic inequities in vaccine hesitancy among native hawaiians and pacific islanders. Health Equity 2022;6(1): 616–24.

28. Jamal A, Wang R, Wang Z, et al. Vaccination patterns, disparities, and policy among AsianAmericans and Asians living in the USA. Abstract. Lancet Glob Health 2022;10(Special Issue 27):27.

29. Garrison NA. Genomic justice for native americans: impact of the havasupai case on genetic research. Sci Technol Human Values 2013;38(2):201–23.

30. Indian Health Service (HIS). Statistics and reports. Available at: https://www.ihs. gov/epi/immunization-and-vaccine-preventable-diseases/statistics-and-reports/. Accessed October 20, 2022.

31. Lee Rogers R, Powe N. COVID-19 Information sources and misinformation by faith community. Inquiry 2022;59. 469580221081388.

32. National Conference of State Legislatures. States with religious and philosophical exemptions from school immunization requirements. 2022. Available at: https://

www.ncsl.org/research/health/school-immunization-exemption-state-laws.aspx. Accessed September 6, 2022.

33. Ugale JL, Spielvogle H, Spina C, et al. It's like 1998 again": why parents still refuse and delay vaccines. Glob Pediatr Health 2021;8. 2333794X211042331.

34. Centers for Disease Control and Prevention (CDC). Trusted partners help minneapolis somali community get vaccinated. 2021. Available at: https://www.cdc.gov/vaccines/covid-19/health-departments/features/minneapolis-somali-community.html. Accessed August 17, 2022.

35. Hall V, Banerjee E, Kenyon C, et al. Measles outbreak - minnesota april-may 2017. MMWR Morb Mortal Wkly Rep 2017;66(27):713–7.

36. Zucker JR, Rosen JB, Iwamoto M, et al. Consequences of Undervaccination - Measles Outbreak, New York City, 2018-2019. N Engl J Med 2020;382(11): 1009–17.

37. Marye S, Spencer G. A population study of the NYS measles epidemic: Lessons learned. Public Health Nurs 2022. https://doi.org/10.1111/phn.13084.

38. Link-Gelles R, Lutterloh E, Schnabel Ruppert P, et al. Public health response to a case of paralytic poliomyelitis in an unvaccinated person and detection of poliovirus in wastewater - New York, June-August 2022. MMWR Morb Mortal Wkly Rep 2022;71(33):1065–8.

39. Children's Hospital of Philadelphia. Vaccine Ingredients – Fetal Cells. 2021. Available at: https://www.chop.edu/centers-programs/vaccine-education-center/vaccine-ingredients/fetal-tissues. Accessed October 6, 2022.

40. Gastanaduy PA, Budd J, Fisher N, et al. A measles outbreak in an underimmunized amish community in ohio. N Engl J Med 2016;375(14):1343–54.

41. Scott EM, Stein R, Brown MF, et al. Vaccination patterns of the northeast Ohio Amish revisited. Vaccine 2021;39(7):1058–63.

42. Wenger OK, McManus MD, Bower JR, et al. Underimmunization in Ohio's Amish: parental fears are a greater obstacle than access to care. Pediatrics 2011;128(1): 79–85.

43. Plotkin SA, Offit PA, DeStefano F, et al. The science of vaccine safety: summary of meeting at Wellcome Trust. Vaccin 2020;38(8):1869–80.

44. Gerber JS, Offit PA. Vaccines and autism: a tale of shifting hypotheses. Clin Infect Dis 2009;48(4):456–61.

45. Baylor NW, Egan W, Richman P. Aluminum salts in vaccines–US perspective. Vaccine 2002;20(Suppl 3):S18–23.

46. Daley MF, Reifler LM, Glanz JM, et al. Association Between aluminum exposure from vaccines before age 24 months and persistent asthma at age 24 to 59 months. Acad Pediatr 2022. https://doi.org/10.1016/j.acap.2022.08.006.

47. Racine AD. Aluminum adjuvants in childhood vaccines and asthma risk: what do we see? Acad Pediatr 2022. https://doi.org/10.1016/j.acap.2022.08.007.

48. Viswanath K, Bekalu M, Dhawan D, et al. Individual and social determinants of COVID-19 vaccine uptake. BMC Public Health 2021;21(1):818.

49. Willis DE, Schootman M, Shah SK, et al. Parent/guardian intentions to vaccinate children against COVID-19 in the United States. Hum Vaccin Immunother 2022; 18(5):2071078.

50. Funk C, Gramlich J. 10 facts about Americans and coronavirus vaccines. 2021. Available at: https://www.pewresearch.org/fact-tank/2021/09/20/10-facts-about-americans-and-coronavirus-vaccines/. Accessed September 6, 2022.

51. Sencer DJ, Millar JD. Reflections on the 1976 swine flu vaccination program. Emerg Infect Dis 2006;12(1):29–33.

52. Schwartz H. Swine flu fiasco. The New York Times 1976;33.

53. Larson HJ, Gakidou E, Murray CJL. The Vaccine-Hesitant Moment. N Engl J Med Jul 7 2022;387(1):58–65. https://doi.org/10.1056/NEJMra2106441.

54. Salmon DA, Dudley MZ, Glanz JM, et al. Vaccine hesitancy: causes, consequences, and a call to action. Vaccine 2015;33(Suppl 4):D66–71.

55. Schuler CL, Hanley CJ, Coyne-Beasley T. Misconception: human papillomavirus vaccine and infertility. Clin Pediatr (Phila) 2014;53(2):158–65.

56. Kricorian K, Turner K. COVID-19 vaccine acceptance and beliefs among black and hispanic americans. PLoS One 2021;16(8):e0256122.

57. Hernandez ND, Daley EM, Young L, et al. HPV Vaccine recommendations: does a health care provider's gender and ethnicity matter to Unvaccinated Latina college women? Ethn Health 2019;24(6):645–61.

58. Silberner J. Covid-19: how native americans led the way in the US vaccination effort. BMJ 2021;374:n2168.

59. Haroz EE, Kemp CG, O'Keefe VM, et al. Nurturing innovation at the roots: the success of COVID-19 vaccination in american indian and alaska native communities. Am J Public Health 2022;112(3):383–7.

60. Cotton NK, Shim RS. Social determinants of health, structural racism, and the impact on child and adolescent mental health. J Am Acad Child Adolesc Psychiatry 2022. https://doi.org/10.1016/j.jaac.2022.04.020.

61. Muravsky NL, Betesh GM, McCoy RG. Religious doctrine and attitudes toward vaccination in jewish law. J Relig Health 2021. https://doi.org/10.1007/s10943-021-01447-8.

62. Catholic News Agency Staff. Catholic US bishops approve use of COVID-19 vaccines with 'remote connection' to abortion. 2020. Available at: https://www.catholicnewsagency.com/news/46899/catholic-us-bishops-approve-use-of-covid-19-vaccines-with-remote-connection-to-abortion. Accessed August 18, 2022.

63. World Health Organization (WHO). Judicially prohibited and impure substances in foodstuff and drugs. Letter. 2001. Available at: https://www.immunize.org/talking-about-vaccines/porcine.pdf. Accessed August 23, 2022.

64. Alfieri NL, Kusma JD, Heard-Garris N, et al. Parental COVID-19 vaccine hesitancy for children: vulnerability in an urban hotspot. BMC Public Health 2021;21(1):1662.

65. Szilagyi PG, Shah MD, Delgado JR, et al. Parents' Intentions and Perceptions About COVID-19 Vaccination for Their Children: Results From a National Survey. Pediatrics 2021. https://doi.org/10.1542/peds.2021-052335.

Adolescents, Young Adults, and Vaccine Hesitancy

Who and What Drives the Decision to Vaccinate?

Abigail English, JD[a,b,]*, Amy B. Middleman, MD, MSEd, MPH[c]

KEYWORDS

- Adolescents • Consent • Ethics • Law • Vaccine hesitancy • Young adults

KEY POINTS

- Vaccination rates among adolescents and young adults vary by vaccine and have been slow to reach levels close to those of infants and younger children.
- Complex factors—perceptions/knowledge, sociodemographic context, and misinformation—contribute to vaccine hesitancy for the adolescent and young adult age group.
- Parents and adolescents generally agree about the decision whether to vaccinate; healthcare providers have significant influence in the decision process.
- The legal framework for vaccination consent allows young adults to make the decision for themselves; parent consent is generally required but exceptions in law and policy allow minors to consent in some circumstances.

INTRODUCTION

Although vaccines are important for all age groups, issues of vaccine uptake and vaccine hesitancy have particular salience for the adolescent and young adult age group. This article reviews the importance of vaccination for adolescents and young adults, the variability in uptake of different vaccines, the reasons for vaccine hesitancy for this age group, and the legal framework for consent for vaccination.

IMPORTANCE OF VACCINATION

The importance of vaccination for primary prevention of infectious disease among human beings of all ages cannot be overstated. Development of vaccines is among the 10 most important public health achievements in the United States in the twentieth

[a] Center for Adolescent Health & the Law, PO Box 3795, Chapel Hill, NC 27515, USA; [b] Gillings School of Global Publlic Health, University of North Carolina, Chapel Hill; [c] Department of Pediatrics, University of Oklahoma Health Sciences Center, 1200 Children's Avenue, Suite 12200, Oklahoma City, OK 73104, USA
* Corresponding author. Center for Adolescent Health & the Law, PO Box 3795, Chapel Hill, NC 27515.
E-mail address: abigail.english.cahl@gmail.com

Pediatr Clin N Am 70 (2023) 283–295
https://doi.org/10.1016/j.pcl.2022.11.006
0031-3955/23/© 2022 Elsevier Inc. All rights reserved.

century.[1] Historically in the United States, immunization recommendations targeted infants and children. In 1996, the Centers for Disease Control and Prevention (CDC) created an immunization platform for ages 11 to 12 years, using the Td booster and "catch-up" hepatitis B vaccine as its anchors.[2] More vaccines are now recommended for adolescents and young adults because we are moving toward primary prevention of infectious diseases across the life span. In large part, due to the effectiveness of vaccines, infectious disease is not currently a top 10 cause of mortality among children and adolescents in the United States;[3] preventing disease with vaccination has a very high success rate and, when utilized, is an easy win against morbidity for adolescents.

VACCINE UPTAKE IN ADOLESCENTS AND YOUNG ADULTS

Vaccination rates among adolescents and young adults have been slow to reach levels close to those of infants and children for many reasons. One key reason is that adolescents do not access care as frequently as infants and children; they also have fewer preventive health-care visits. Young adults use office-based care at even lower rates than adolescents.[4]

Multiple factors contribute to reduced opportunities for health-care interventions with adolescents and young adults. As children enter adolescence, their developmental tasks shift toward separation and individuation from parents and guardians. They are busy creating independent identities, they can transport themselves, and they are less likely to do all they are asked to do. Prevention may seem less compelling if they perceive the risk of spending time away from higher stakes academic pursuits or activities with peers as more important than seeking preventive health care that may yield benefits far in the future. Adolescents' own schedules get busy, and busy parents may not remember adolescent immunization timelines.

The decision to vaccinate an adolescent is no longer solely within the purview of the parent; the adolescent also has input. Adolescents and young adults often look to their parents for health-care advice and usually agree with their parents on decisions regarding vaccination[5–8] but their fear of needles and concerns about vaccine side effects disrupting other activities can delay vaccination.

Vaccination Rates for Specific Vaccines

Rates of vaccination also differ based on the specific vaccine being considered. The vaccines now recommended for adolescents include Tdap, HPV, and MenACWY vaccines at age 11 to 12 years, and MenACWY and MenB vaccines at age 16 years. Influenza vaccine is routinely recommended annually, and COVID-19 vaccination recommendations continue to evolve. Vaccination rates among adolescents have slowly increased over time. Per the National Immunization Survey – Teen (NIS-Teen) for the year 2021,[9] the national rate of vaccination among those ages 13 to 17 years was as follows:

- Tdap: 89.6%
- HPV
  - 76.9% for at least one dose
  - 61.7% for up-to-date HPV vaccination status
- MenACWY
  - 89.0% for at least one dose
  - 60.0% for at least 2 doses
- MenB: 31.4%

The grossly lower rate of vaccination for MenB vaccine is likely secondary to MenB vaccine's shared clinical decision-making recommendation—a recommendation that emphasizes discussion and vaccine decision-making based on patient circumstances and goals rather than a recommendation that should be applied to all adolescents.[10] Rates of influenza vaccination have recently been approximately 50% to 60% among children and adolescents aged 1 to 17 years.[10] Despite similar years of introduction and same age of recommended administration of the first dose, rates of vaccination of at least 1 MenACWY vaccine, first recommended in 2005, significantly exceed rates of at least 1 dose of HPV vaccine, first recommended for female adolescents in 2006 (the dosing interval for series completion differs too greatly for valid comparison). Even when looking specifically at female rates of at least 1 dose of HPV vaccination because this was the first group for whom the vaccine was recommended (78.5%), MenACWY vaccination rates have enjoyed far greater success.

REASONS FOR VACCINE HESITANCY

The differences in vaccination rates—and hesitancy—for different vaccines represent a complex constellation of considerations including:

- Perceptions/knowledge about the target disease including disease severity and judgment regarding mode of transmission
- Perceptions/knowledge about the available vaccines
- Available delivery systems
- Sociodemographic and cultural context of the patient

These factors also play a role in vaccine prioritization among patients, parents, and providers.

Perceptions and Knowledge Related to Diseases Targeted by Vaccines

The Tdap recommendation in 2005 generated little fanfare. The diseases against which the vaccine provides protection had well-known names; Tdap essentially replaced Td in the schedule for children aged 11 and 12 years, and pertussis vaccine has been given to children at a younger age for many decades. There was little controversy, and all states now require Tdap for school attendance.

Introduction of MenACWY in 2005 was not quite as smooth. Fewer people were familiar with the disease; it took time to educate parents regarding the disease and to overcome initial supply concerns related to unanticipated use outside of the initially recommended age recommendations. The threat of meningitis is frightening to most people; the disease is relatively uncommon but the potential devastation resulting from the disease prompts action. With increased communication about the hazards of the disease itself as well as an increasing number of states requiring the vaccine for school, rates of vaccination against meningitis have slowly but steadily increased.

Response to the recommendation for the HPV vaccine for adolescents was surprisingly complex in the United States. The HPV vaccine is the second vaccine released that serves as a prevention of cancer (hepatitis B vaccine was the first). It prevents acquisition of the virus that causes cervical, vaginal, and vulvar cancers; penile and anal cancers; and head and neck cancers with efficacy of greater than 90%.[11] Primary preventive strategies for cancer have been eagerly awaited for years but the HPV vaccine became controversial largely based on the mode of transmission of the target disease (**Box 1**). (See Daisy Y. Morales-Campos, and colleagues' article "Human Papillomavirus Vaccine Hesitancy in the United States," in this issue) Clinicians can help patients and parents focus on disease prevention and discourage distractions based on misinformation or unrelated details in their recommendations for vaccination.

> **Box 1**
> **HPV vaccine: a lesson learned?**
>
> HPV is primarily a sexually transmitted virus. The fact that the HPV vaccine prevents disease and future cancer was overshadowed by concern about whether children were engaging in sex. Acceptability among providers and parents was less for younger than for older adolescents.[21–23] Public messaging failed *first* to convey the primary importance of stopping the disease with the effective means available and *then* to address the specific behavior of adolescents—a much more difficult task—as a distinctly separate issue. Rates of vaccination series completion among adolescents aged 13 to 17 years with this highly successful vaccine have just reached more than 60% in 2021, even after the number of doses required for series completion for healthy adolescents under 15 years of age dropped from 3 to 2 in 2016.[25] Moreover, providers significantly underestimate parents' valuation of the HPV vaccine for adolescents.[26] Because provider recommendation is the most important factor in determining vaccine acceptance,[27–30] a disconnect between parent and provider communication and missed opportunities for education have likely played a significant role in vaccine hesitancy related to the HPV vaccine.

Perception and Knowledge Related to Specific Vaccines

Although the decision to receive a specific vaccine may be affected by perceptions associated with the target disease, issues related to the vaccine itself can also become a reason to avoid or delay vaccination. There are those who are concerned about thimerosal (now found only in multidose vials of flu vaccine), various adjuvants, and use of fetal cells in vaccine development—none of which are associated with harm. Misinformation related to vaccine side effects for adolescents has been circulating since the hepatitis B vaccine was recommended for adolescents in the 1990s. When the vaccine was first released for use among adolescents, there were reports of hair loss, fatigue, and multiple sclerosis because of vaccination. These concerns were later quelled with research.[31]

By the time the HPV vaccine was released, social media were a common source of information for adolescents and families. The HPV vaccine was met not only with concerns about side effects but also with misinformation such as claims by politicians that the vaccine caused "mental retardation."[32] Although it is not always clear who benefits from this type of misinformation, anti-vaccine messaging has the potential to be a profitable commercial business for many people.[45]

Misconceptions often are related to misunderstanding of the safety protections in place after a vaccine is released to the market. Although safety is studied prelicensure, the CDC uses multiple vaccine safety systems postlicensure. The most recognized is the Vaccine Adverse Event Reporting System (VAERS). Few people understand that issues signaled by VAERS data—data that are publicly available—have not yet been rigorously studied (**Box 2**). Even fewer people are aware of the Vaccine Safety Datalink and the Clinical Immunization Safety Assessment Project that both allow for rigorous, ongoing monitoring, and proactive clinical research on vaccine safety. Becoming more familiar with the safety programs in place to protect patients and families may help providers more confidently recommend lifesaving vaccines.

Delivery Systems and Social Context: Examining COVID-19 Vaccine

The story of the most recently released vaccine, the COVID-19 vaccine, includes nearly all of the multifaceted plot elements that lead to vaccine hesitancy. Many of these factors have been important in the evolving rollout of the COVID-19 vaccine for adolescents and young adults.

> **Box 2**
> **Strengths and weaknesses of VAERS**
>
> VAERS is a passive reporting system, designed to gather information from anyone and everyone in order to look for any patterns—or signals–related to vaccine side effects and adverse events. It is also a public reporting system; anyone can report problems (a young patient's second cousin twice removed could report a suspected vaccine side effect) and the list of these reported events is available to the public. Often, those quoting VAERS data fail to acknowledge that the adverse events reported may not have been verified and are not necessarily causally related to vaccination.[46] A young person could experience death by alcohol intoxication several hours after getting vaccinated, and it would be registered in VAERS as a death temporally related to vaccination; however, there is no causal relationship between the death and the vaccination.

There has been misinformation related to the disease and its severity. Although the risk of severe disease is lower among children and adolescents than older adults after contracting COVID-19 disease, from January 1, 2020 to May 11, 2022, 443 deaths from COVID-19 among adolescents aged 12 to 17 years had been reported to the CDC.[47] The disease accounts for 2.4% of deaths in this age group.[47] Many more have been hospitalized, and hospitalization rates are significantly lower among those who have been vaccinated.[47] With COVID-19, as with most diseases, young people also serve as vectors for infectious disease.

Misinformation about COVID-19 and the vaccine have been propagated not only by antivaccine groups but also by politicians. Although the twenty-first century has seen vaccination rates become increasingly associated with political affiliation,[48] COVID-19 disease and vaccination has become one of the most flagrantly politicized vaccination issues in recent history—all the way to the Office of the President. Messages on social media played an increasingly important role throughout the pandemic; a higher proportion of teens and parents reported concerns regarding what they were reading on social media about the safety of vaccines as the pandemic wore on.[5] There were also concerns with the new vaccination platform (mRNA technology). Vaccination rates among adolescents aged 12 to 17 years reached 60.5% as of August 31, 2022;[49] however, rates still differ based on sociodemographic factors including ethnicity (more Hispanic adolescents are vaccinated than non-Hispanic) and community type (more adolescents in urban and suburban areas are vaccinated than in rural areas).[47] More adolescents were vaccinated with COVID-19 vaccine outside of the medical home than with any other vaccine in recent years due to the need for speedy and efficient delivery; 48% of adolescents aged 12 to 17 years were vaccinated in a pharmacy.[47] Interestingly, during the course of the pandemic, attitudes regarding the disease and intention to vaccinate changed little both for parents of adolescents and for adolescents themselves; attitudes and vaccination patterns of adolescents and their parents were significantly aligned.[5] Vaccination rates may improve as clinicians further understand messaging that will help address the unique patient/parent concerns and access issues within the specific communities they serve.

WHO MAKES THE DECISION TO VACCINATE?

One important difference between vaccine hesitancy for adolescents and hesitancy for younger children or adults is the unique developmental, clinical, ethical, and legal context in which the decision to vaccinate is made.[50] The legal baseline is that for adolescent minors, aged younger than 18 years, parent consent is generally required but state minor consent laws may create exceptions. Adolescents who are young adults, aged 18 years or older, are allowed to consent for themselves.

Vaccine Decision Process

As noted above, independent of who has the legal authority, the dynamic relationship between adolescents and their parents is a key element in adolescent vaccination; this dynamic is also influenced by the health-care provider.[51] Parents and adolescents influence each other in the process of deciding whether or not an adolescent will receive a particular vaccine. The adolescent–parent dynamic also is influenced by many factors including the evolving capacity of the adolescent to make decisions as well as the legal framework.

Concordance or discordance within the parent–adolescent dyad may affect vaccine hesitancy in varied ways. The parent may be hesitant and the adolescent eager, or conversely, the parent may be eager and the adolescent reluctant. Both may be eager, or both may be hesitant. Each of these situations require different skilled responses from the adolescent's health-care provider—to educate, counsel, and support in ways that preferably lead to a decision with which all parties are comfortable. The specific content of public health educational messages and individual counseling should be crafted with consideration of the sources and reasons for the parent and/or adolescent's vaccine hesitancy (see "Clinicals Care Points" section).

Recent research on COVID-19 vaccination looked at parents' perspectives with respect to how often they considered their adolescents' desires and how they perceived concordance and discordance between their own preferences and the desires of the adolescents.[52] Almost three-fifths—58%—of parents considered their adolescents' desires; those who did so were more likely to vaccinate.[52] The same proportion—nearly three-fifths—perceived concordance between their own desires and those of their adolescents; only 2.4% perceived discordance, with the adolescent desiring vaccination and the parent not willing to vaccinate.[52]

Before the COVID-19 pandemic, a study of young adolescents in middle school found that more than half perceived that vaccination decisions were made by their parents and the doctor; one-third by parents and adolescent together.[53] More than half thought their mothers had the biggest influence on whether they were vaccinated; about one-third thought the doctor had the biggest influence. Similar proportions—about 30%—wanted the doctor to decide, wanted their parent to decide, or wanted to decide for themselves.[53] These studies, along with other research, suggest the importance of involving youth in the decision to vaccinate.

Not only are parental influences important for adolescents who are minors but also for adolescents who are young adults. For clinicians, this underscores the need to educate both patients and parents whenever possible, even when the patients are aged older than 18 years. Many young adults continue to share health information with their parents, seek their advice about health care, and are influenced by their parents' views and behaviors.[54] This pattern may persist with the decision whether or not to be vaccinated. When young adults disagree with their parents, they can make the decision themselves. When adolescent minors disagree, the legal framework for vaccination consent must be considered (**Box 3**).

Legal Framework for Vaccination Consent

Consent for vaccination for adolescents takes place in the broader context of consent for health care generally. Consent requirements are determined primarily by

> **Box 3**
> **COVID-19 focuses attention on adolescent consent for vaccination**
>
> During the COVID-19 pandemic, as vaccines became available and were authorized for the adolescent age group, increased attention focused on the question of whether and when adolescent minors should be allowed to give their own consent for vaccination. This type of attention was not new; it had also risen during a recent outbreak of measles.[55] Medical organizations also had previously issued opinions offering support for minors to be able to consent for vaccination.[56–58] During the COVID-19 pandemic health policy researchers identified patterns in current policies;[56] a plethora of lawyers, medical ethicists, health policy experts, and journalists provided analysis and recommendations.[59–61,12–16] These recent perspectives shed light on a longstanding issue that may continue to require attention as new infectious diseases emerge and pandemics develop.

state laws, which vary from state to state. Health-care providers must understand the legal framework for consent for health care in their state. For adolescents who are minors, aged younger than 18 years, parent consent is usually required. Alternatives to parent consent include consent by legal guardians, and sometimes by other adults who have custody of an adolescent and have been granted legal authority to consent. When youth are in state custody—in foster care or the juvenile justice system—parents may retain authority to consent. Courts also may have authority to grant consent for health care, or it may be delegated to a child welfare agency or other government official. Although states often do not have explicit laws requiring parent consent for vaccination, the general rule would apply unless there is a relevant exception. When parents legally may consent for an adolescent minor's vaccination, it is nevertheless clinically and ethically important to obtain the adolescent's assent.

Every state has laws defining the circumstances in which adolescent minors may consent for their own health care.[17,18] Some of these exceptions are relevant for vaccination.[50] Adolescent minors may be able consent for health care because they have a particular status or living situation or because they are seeking a specific service.

Groups of minors who may be able to consent for all or most of their own health care in one or more states include the following:

- Minors who have reached a specific age such as 15 or 16 years
- Minors legally emancipated by court order
- Minors who meet certain criteria of maturity such as having the capacity to give informed consent
- Minors who live apart from their parents and may be homeless
- Married minors
- Minor parents (for themselves and/or their child)
- Minors in active military service
- Incarcerated minors

Not all states have laws covering each of these categories. However, if authorized by state law to consent for their own health care, these minors would be able to consent for vaccination as well as other services.

Some or all states allow adolescent minors to give their own consent for a wide array of services including several sexual and reproductive health services, as well as care related to mental health and substance use.[17,18] Not all of these laws would necessarily authorize an adolescent minor to consent for vaccination. Laws directly related to the following services might encompass vaccination:

- Vaccination (generally or for specific diseases or conditions such as hepatitis B, HPV, or COVID-19)
- Prevention, diagnosis, and/or treatment of sexually transmitted disease or infection or venereal disease
- Prevention, diagnosis, and/or treatment of infectious, contagious, communicable, or reportable disease.[18–20]

A law that authorizes an adolescent minor to consent for *"diagnosis and treatment"* of sexually transmitted infections or infectious diseases would not necessarily allow them to consent for vaccination unless it had been interpreted to do so. When *"prevention"* is included, an adolescent minor should be able to consent for vaccination. In some states, adolescent minors are allowed to consent to a specific vaccine but not to other vaccines.

A small number of states have had laws such as this in place for many years; a few others have more recently enacted statutes or issued policies—or considered doing so—to create such authority.[18–20] Whether an adolescent minor is allowed to give their own consent for a vaccination depends on several factors:

- Specific vaccine and specific disease for which it is administered
- State or local jurisdiction where vaccination will take place
- Specific status of minor (eg, married or emancipated)
- Age of minor
- Capacity of minor to give informed consent

These factors, considered in the context of state or local laws and policies, must be carefully analyzed to determine whether an adolescent minor is authorized to consent for vaccination in a specific situation.

Consent Considerations in Specific Health Care Settings

Adolescents and young adults receive health care, including vaccinations, in a wide variety of health-care settings that are funded by varied federal, state, and local sources.[24] A few of these settings are subject to special regulations or policies that may affect the vaccination decision. Two such settings of particular importance are family planning clinics and school-based health centers (SBHCs).

In many communities, family planning clinics exist either as freestanding sites or operate as part of hospital ambulatory care systems, public health departments, federally qualified health centers (FQHCs), or other health systems. In most of these sites, the same consent rules would apply as in other health-care settings. However, family planning services that are funded by the federal Title X Family Planning Program are subject to specific rules.[33,34] Title X funded sites are permitted to offer "preventive health services that are considered beneficial to reproductive health such as HPV vaccination."[35] The Title X regulations provide that parental consent may not be required; notification of parents is not permitted without the permission of the minor.[36]

SBHCs are another venue in which many adolescents and some young adults receive health care, including vaccinations. SBHCs operate under the auspices of school districts, health departments, health systems and hospitals, and FQHCs; some receive Title X funding. In most SBHCs, the consent laws of the state in which they are located apply. However, SBHCs also generally have specific policies governing what is required for a student to enroll in the center and receive services. The consent forms vary among SBHCs; often the applicable policies are determined by the school district or health department, depending on the auspices under which the

SBHC is operating. Parental consent to use the services is almost always required for adolescent minors; young adults would be able to enroll independently. Some consent forms allow parents to "opt-in" or "opt-out" for their adolescent to receive specific services: sometimes the policy specifies that minors are allowed to consent and receive services confidentially consistent with applicable state and federal laws.[37,38]

PUBLIC POLICY RESPONSES

Efforts to increase vaccine uptake among adolescents and young adults and overcome vaccine hesitancy for this population have included many public policy responses. Notable among them are vaccine mandates, communication strategies, and improvements to the public health infrastructure.

Vaccine mandates have been put in place as school and college entry requirements and as conditions of employment in certain settings. The rationales for mandates related to vaccines for different diseases in different settings have been based, variously, on the disease's transmissibility; the setting as an opportunity for transmission, or risk of transmission; or the potential for significant public health disruption or cost. Particularly in recent years, substantial controversies have arisen regarding vaccine mandates as well as the scope of exemptions, especially with respect to certain vaccines. Initial efforts to incorporate HPV vaccine into school entry requirements foundered; and even longstanding mandates, such as for measles, encountered opposition; so did recent requirements for COVID-19 vaccination. Policies allowing exemptions for medical reasons and for religious or personal beliefs have been evolving in an arena increasingly characterized by both vaccine-related controversies and public health threats.[39] This is unfortunate; the effectiveness of vaccine mandates in increasing vaccination rates is well established.[40–42] Indeed, rates of vaccination with nonrequired vaccines among adolescents have been shown to increase when other adolescent vaccines are mandated; a 2010 report documented a nearly 5% increased initiation of HPV vaccine (42.9% vs 47.3%; $P = .004$) in states that had enacted mandates for Td/Tdap vaccine.[43]

Devising the most effective communication strategies—public health guidance and community outreach and education—for increasing vaccine uptake and overcoming hesitancy is especially challenging for the adolescent and young adult population. Part of the challenge has to do with the need to reach both adolescents and their parents, who receive and respond to messaging in different ways. Moreover, in recent years and especially during the COVID-19 pandemic, the dominant influence of the Internet, social media, and online forms of information, misinformation, and disinformation has complicated the task even further. (See Todd Wolynn, and colleagues' article "Social Media and Vaccine Hesitancy," in this issue)

In this context, generating youth-centered materials to address adolescents' concerns directly and provide assurances of safety and rationales for recommended vaccination is an important approach. This is not only helpful for patients and parents but clinicians strongly value having such educational materials available for themselves and patients.[44] Other related approaches might include better use by public health entities or media-trained providers of social media to refute misinformation and working with youth as social media influencers and ambassadors to their peers.

Finally, improving the public health infrastructure in ways that expand opportunities targeted at the adolescent age group may be an effective strategy. Increasing the availability of vaccination at schools and alternative sites is one potentially effective way of doing that.

SUMMARY

Vaccine hesitancy among adolescents and young adults is complex due to multiple factors: their developmental stage, the psychosocial and demographic context, the dynamic relationship in the adolescent–parent dyad, access to information and misinformation, accessibility of vaccines, and the legal framework that allows or disallows them to consent or assent to receive vaccines. Health-care providers are uniquely positioned to improve adolescent immunization rates by influencing the vaccination decision and advocating for ways to overcome vaccine hesitancy and other barriers for this age group. Ultimately, providing adolescent and young adult patients and their parents with evidence-based information to support them in making the decision affords maximal benefit in the process.

CLINICAL CARE POINTS

- Provider recommendation is the most important factor in family decisions about whether an adolescent or young adult will be vaccinated. Address both the patient and their parent/guardian.
- Be prepared for vaccine conversations with patients and families with 2 or 3 relevant facts pertaining to
  - The vaccine-preventable disease itself
  - The vaccine(s) available to prevent the disease (including safety and efficacy)
  - The reasons patients should get vaccinated
- Prepare messages designed to reach adolescents and young adults as well as parents.
- Directly refute vaccine myths with facts. Recommend the CDC.gov or immunize.org websites for further information.
- Know the laws in your state related to circumstances in which minors are allowed to consent to receive vaccines.
- When an adolescent minor is independently seeking vaccination, consider
  - Specific vaccine being sought
  - Status and age of minor
  - Capacity of minor to give informed consent

DISCLOSURE

A. English receives royalty payments from WoltersKluwer as a section editor for UpToDate. Middleman's institution entered into a service agreement within the past 24 months with Pfizer for research regarding shared clinical decision-making and the MenB vaccine; A.B. Middleman served as the principal investigator. A.B. Middleman receives royalty payments from WoltersKluwer as an author and a section editor for UpToDate.

REFERENCES

1. CDC. Ten great public health achievements—United States, 1900-1999. MMWR 1999;48(12):241–3.
2. CDC. Immunization of adolescents: recommendations of the advisory committee on immunization practices, the American Academy of Pediatrics, the American Academy of Family Physicians, and the American Medical Association. MMWR 1996;45(No. RR-13):1–16.

3. Goldstick JE, Cunningham RM, Carter PM. Current causes of death in children and adolescents in the United States. N Engl J Med 2022;386(20):1955–6.
4. Lau JS, Adams SH, Boscardin WJ, et al. Young adults' health care utilization and expenditures prior to the Affordable Care Act. J Adolesc Health 2014;54(6): 663–71.
5. Middleman AB, Klein J, Quinn J. Vaccine hesitancy in the time of COVID-19: attitudes and intentions of teens and parents regarding the COVID-19 vaccine. Vaccines (Basel) 2021;10(1):4.
6. Painter JE, Gargano LM, Sales JM, et al. Correlates of 2009 H1N1 influenza vaccine acceptability among parents and their adolescent children. Health Educ Res 2011;26(5):751–60.
7. Rosenthal SL, Kottenhahn RK, Biro FM, et al. Hepatitis B vaccine acceptance among adolescents and their parents. J Adolesc Health 1995;17(4):248–54.
8. Zimet GD, Perkins SM, Sturm LA, et al. Predictors of STI vaccine acceptability among parents and their adolescent children. J Adolesc Health 2005;37 (3): 179–86.
9. Pingali C, Yankey D, Elam-Evans LD, et al. National vaccination coverage among adolescents aged 13-17 years—National Immunization Survey-Teen, United States, 2021. MMWR 2022;71:1101–8.
10. CDC. QuickStats: percentage of children and adolescents aged 1–17 years who received an influenza vaccine within the past 12 months, by health insurance coverage and age group—National Health Interview Survey, United States, 2019–2020. MMWR 2021;70:1785.
11. Markowitz LE, Schiller JT. Human papillomavirus vaccines. J Infect Dis 2021; 224(12 Suppl 2):S367–78.
12. McCave EL. Influential factors in HPV vaccination uptake among providers in four states. J Community Health 2010;35(6):645–52.
13. Gerend MA, Weibley E, Bland H. Parental response to human papillomavirus vaccine availability: uptake and intentions. J Adolesc Health 2009;45:528–31.
14. Kahn JA, Ding L, Huang B, et al. Mothers' intention for their daughters and themselves to receive the human papillomavirus vaccine: a national study of nurses. Pediatrics 2009;123:1439–45.
15. Meites E, Kempe A, Markowitz LE. Use of a 2-dose schedule for human papillomavirus vaccination — updated recommendations of the Advisory Committee on Immunization Practices. MMWR 2016;65:1405–8.
16. Healy CM, Montesinos DP, Middleman AB. Parent and provider perspectives on immunization: are providers overestimating parental concerns? Vaccine 2014; 32(5):579–84.
17. Gust DA, Darling N, Kennedy A, et al. Parents with doubts about vaccines: which vaccines and reasons why. Pediatrics 2008;122:718–25.
18. Dorell C, Yankey D, Kennedy A, et al. Factors that influence parental vaccination decisions for adolescents, 13 to 17 years old: National Immunization Survey—Teen. Clin Pediatr 2013;52:162–70.
19. Gust DA, Kennedy A, Shui I, et al. Parent attitudes toward immunizations and healthcare providers: the role of information. Am J Prev Med 2005;29:105–12.
20. Smith PJ, Kennedy A, Wooten K, et al. Association between health care providers' influence on parents who have concerns about vaccine safety and vaccination coverage. Pediatrics 2006;118(5):e1287–92.
21. Zuckerman JN. Protective efficacy, immunotherapeutic potential, and safety of hepatitis B vaccines. J Med Virol 2006;78(2):169–77.

22. Harper M., The Gardasil problem: how the U.S. lost faith in a promising vaccine, 2012, Forbes, Available at: https://www.forbes.com/sites/matthewherper/2012/04/04/americas-gardasil-problem-how-politics-poisons-public-health/?sh=54154fae5c27. Accessed October 15, 2022.
23. Whyte L.E., The center for public integrity. spreading vaccine fears, Available at: https://publicintegrity.org/?s=spreading%20fears%20cashing%20in%20, 2021. Accessed October 15, 2022.
24. Shimabukuro TT, Nguyen M, Martin D, et al. Safety monitoring in the vaccine adverse event reporting system (VAERS). Vaccine 2015;33(36):4398–405.
25. Oliver S., Evidence to Recommendation (EtR) Framework: Moderna COVID-19 vaccine in children ages 6 –11 years and adolescents ages 12 –17 years, ACIP Meeting, June 23, 2022.
26. Bernstein S, North A, Schwartz J, et al. State-level voting patterns and adolescent vaccination coverage in the United States, 2014. Am J Public Health 2016; 106(10):1879–81.
27. CDC, COVID data tracker, Available at: https://covid.cdc.gov/covid-data-tracker/#vaccinations_vacc-people-additional-dose-totalpop. Accessed October 15, 2022.
28. English A, Shaw MD, McCauley MM, et al. Legal basis of consent for health care and vaccination for adolescents. Pediatrics 2008;121(Supp1):S85–7.
29. Limaye RJ, Opel DJ, Dempsey A, et al. Communicating with vaccine-hesitant parents: a narrative review. Acad Pediatr 2021;21(4):S24–9.
30. Delgado JF, Szilagyi PG, Peralta JB, et al. Influence of perceived adolescent vaccination desire on parent decision for adolescent COVID-19 vaccination. J Adolesc Health 2022;70:567–70.
31. Herman R, McNutt LA, Mehta M, et al. Vaccination perspectives among adolescents and their desired role in the decision-making process. Hum Vaccin Immunother 2019;15:1752–9.
32. Sandler K, Srivastava T, Fawole OA, et al. Understanding vaccine knowledge attitudes, and decision-making through college student interviews. J Am Coll Health 2020;68(6):593–602.
33. Yang YT, Olick RS, Shaw J. Adolescent consent to vaccination in the age of vaccine-hesitant parents. JAMA Pediatr 2019;173(12):1123–4.
34. Matshazi N. AMA backs states allowing 'mature minors' to consent to vaccinations. Healthcare Weekly June 21, 2019.
35. English A, Ford CA, Kahn JA, et al. Adolescent consent for vaccination: a position paper of the Society for Adolescent Health and Medicine. J Adolesc Health 2013; 53:550–3.
36. Singer N., Kates J. and Tolbert J., Kaiser Family Foundation. COVID-19 vaccination and parental consent, Available at: https://www.kff.org/policy-watch/covid-19-vaccination-and-parental-consent/, 2021. Accessed October 15, 2022.
37. Agrawal S, Morain SR. Who calls the shots? The ethics of adolescent self-consent for HPV vaccination. J Med Ethics 2018;44(8):531–5.
38. Hoff T. and Kao A., Ethics talk: should adolescents be able to consent for COVID-19 vaccinations?, Available at: https://journalofethics.ama-assn.org/videocast/ethics-talk-should-adolescents-be-able-consent-covid-19-vaccinations, AMA Journal of Ethics, July 27, 2021. Accessed October 15, 2022.
39. Hoffman J., As parents forbid Covid shots, defiant teenagers seek ways to get them. The New York Times, Available at: https://www.nytimes.com/2021/06/26/health/covid-vaccine-teens-consent.html, 2021. Accessed October 15, 2022.

40. McGrew S, Taylor HA. Adolescents, parents, and Covid-19 vaccination—who should decide? NEJM 2022;386(2):e2.
41. Morgan L., Schwartz JL, Sisti DA. COVID-19 vaccination of minors without parental consent: respecting emerging autonomy and advancing public health. JAMA Pediatr 2021;175(10):995–6.
42. Mubarak E, Firn J. When parents don't want their teenager to be vaccinated against COVID-19, who calls the shots? Am J Bioethics 2022;22(1):66–8.
43. Olick RS, Yang YT, Shaw J. Adolescent consent to COVID-19 vaccination: the need for law reform. Pub Health Rep 2022;137(1):163–7.
44. Weithorn LA, Reiss DR. Providing adolescents with independent and confidential access to childhood vaccines: a proposal to lower the age of consent. Conn Law Rev 2020;52:771–861.
45. English A, Bass L, Boyle A, et al. State minor consent laws: a summary. 3rd edition. Chapel Hill (NC): Center for Adolescent Health & the Law; 2010.
46. Sharko M, Jameson R, Ancker JS, et al. State-by-state variability in adolescent privacy laws. Pediatrics 2022;149(6). e2021053458.
47. Zimet GD, Silverman RD, Bednarczyk RA, et al. Adolescent consent for Human Papillomavirus vaccine: ethical, legal, and practical considerations. J Pediatr 2021;231:24–30.
48. Mihaly L.K., Schapiro N.A. and English A., From Human Papillomavirus to COVID-19: adolescent autonomy and minor consent for vaccines, *J Pediatr Health Care*, 36 (6), 2022, 607-610.
49. Hofstetter AM, Schaffer S. Childhood and adolescent vaccination in alternative settings. Acad Pediatr 2021;21(4):S50–6.
50. 42 U.S.C. §§ 300 et seq.
51. C.F.R. Part, 59.
52. Office of Population Affairs U.S. Department of Health and Human Services. Title X Family Planning Program, Available at: https://opa.hhs.gov/sites/default/files/2021-01/HHS-OPA-Title-X-Family-Planning-Program_0.pdf. Accessed October 15, 2022.
53. 42 C.F.R. § 59.10(b).
54. National Conference of State Legislatures. School-Based Health Centers, Available at: https://www.ncsl.org/portals/1/documents/health/HRSBHC.pdf, 2011. Accessed October 15, 2022.
55. Pan RJ. Political will, vaccines, and community immunity. Acad Pediatr 2021; 21(4):S65–6.
56. Lawler EC. Effectiveness of vaccine recommendations versus mandates: evidence from the hepatitis A vaccine. J Health Econ 2017;52:45–62.
57. National Vaccine Advisory Committee. Mandates for adolescent immunizations: recommendations from the National Vaccine Advisory Committee. Am J Prev Med 2008;35:145–51.
58. Bugenske E, Stokley S, Kennedy A, et al. Middle school vaccination requirements and adolescent vaccination coverage. Pediatrics 2012;129(6):1056–63.
59. Dempsey AF, Schaffer SE. Human papillomavirus vaccination rates and state mandates for tetanus-containing vaccines. Prev Med 2011;52:268–9.
60. Middleman AB, Zimet GD, Srivastava AK, et al. Making a shared decision on meningococcal b vaccine: provider feedback on an educational tool developed for use with patients. Acad Pediatr 2022;22(4):564–72.
61. Daley MF, Glanz JM. Using social media to increase vaccine acceptance. Acad Pediatr 2021;21(4):S32–3.

Overcoming Parents' Vaccine Hesitancy

Using Technology to Overcome Vaccine Hesitancy

Francis J. Real, MD, MEd[a,b,*], Matthew W. Zackoff, MD, MEd[a,c],
Brittany L. Rosen, PhD, MEd, CHES®[a,d]

KEYWORDS

- Vaccine hesitancy • Technology • Information systems • Virtual reality
- Mobile apps

KEY POINTS

- Technological innovations are uniquely positioned to address many determinants of vaccine hesitancy and enhance vaccine uptake.
- Patient/parent and provider-level interventions using technology to support vaccine education should align with adult-learning and behavior-change theories.
- Interventions aiming to increase vaccine uptake through technology should include components specifically targeting providers' skills related to addressing vaccine hesitancy.
- Increased accessibility to the Internet, smartphones, and immersive technologies such as virtual reality provide novel avenues to address determinants of vaccine hesitancy.

INTRODUCTION: THE ROLE OF TECHNOLOGY TO ADDRESS VACCINE HESITANCY

In 2019, the World Health Organization (WHO) declared vaccine hesitancy, defined as "delay in acceptance or refusal of vaccination despite availability of vaccination services," a top 10 threat to global health.[1,2] Such hesitancy might impair our ability to effectively curtail infectious diseases such as COVID-19 which negatively impact global health.[3] Thus, a specific Working Group within the Strategic Advisory Group of Experts on Immunizations, an organization charged with advising the WHO on vaccine policies, identified key determinants that related to vaccine hesitancy.[2] These determinants included contextual factors (eg, media, historical influences, perception of pharmaceutical industry), individual and group influences (eg, knowledge, awareness, perceived risk/benefit, trust of health system and providers,

[a] Department of Pediatrics, University of Cincinnati College of Medicine, 3230 Eden Avenue, Cincinnati, OH, USA; [b] Division of General and Community Pediatrics, Cincinnati Children's Hospital Medical Center, 3333 Burnet Avenue, Cincinnati, OH, USA; [c] Division of Critical Care Medicine, Cincinnati Children's Hospital Medical Center, 3333 Burnet Avenue, Cincinnati, OH, USA; [d] Division of Adolescent and Transition Medicine, Cincinnati Children's Hospital Medical Center, 3333 Burnet Avenue, Cincinnati, OH, USA
* Corresponding author. 3333 Burnet Avenue, MLC 2011, Cincinnati, OH 45229.
E-mail address: francis.real@cchmc.org

Pediatr Clin N Am 70 (2023) 297–308
https://doi.org/10.1016/j.pcl.2022.11.007
pediatric.theclinics.com

vaccination as a social norm), and vaccine-specific issues (eg, introduction of a new vaccine, vaccination program design, strength of health care provider recommendation). More recently, the Measuring Behavioral and Social Drivers of Vaccination global expert panel has provided a conceptual model related to vaccine uptake with the following domains: thinking and feeling, social processes, motivation, and practical factors.[4,5]

Several strategies to address vaccine hesitancy determinants and enhance vaccine uptake have been implemented with variable success. Examples include patient reminder systems, provider prompts, brief behavioral interventions, and training plus feedback.[6] In an attempt to increase intervention effectiveness, recent trials have incorporated technology to a greater degree. Technology holds tremendous potential to support up-to-date vaccination status in patients as it is uniquely positioned to amplify positive vaccine messages, support patients and parents' vaccine knowledge, and enhance providers' recommendation skills. Technology may address particular vaccine hesitancy determinants through such modalities as automated reminder systems, integrated decision support for clinicians, online education, social media, and virtual reality (VR).[7] Moreover, the near ubiquitous access to the Internet and smartphones allows for the utilization of technological interventions by a broad range of patients, parents, and providers even among vulnerable, financially insecure populations.[8]

Our aim was to synthesize the best available evidence regarding the use of technology in addressing vaccine hesitancy determinants. This review is organized by the use of (1) hospital and health care center information systems, (2) Web-based information, (3) mobile apps, and (4) VR. These sections are further subcategorized into patient/parent-level interventions and provider-level interventions.

Information Systems

Information systems, such as patient reminder/recall systems and provider clinical decision support, promote childhood vaccination by increasing the frequency and reliability of offering vaccinations. At the patient/parent-level, reminder/recall interventions likely improve vaccination rates by increasing awareness of vaccination status.[9–11] A systematic review of 75 studies found that all assessed types of reminder/recall systems (eg, telephone calls, letters, postcards, text messages, autodialers) were effective in increasing vaccination rates from 5% to 20% points.[11] Person-to-person telephone calls demonstrated the highest level of effectiveness. However, person-to-person telephone calls were also the most costly, with a randomized controlled trial finding that the cost to achieve fully vaccinated status for a single individual was $714.98.[10] A large two-state trial using a centralized autodialer reminder/recall system demonstrated minimal effect on increasing influenza vaccine rates (an absolute difference of 0.6%–1.7% when compared with usual care), though costs were much more modest at approximately $0.20 to 0.30 per participating child.[12] Text messaging offers a low-cost and potentially scalable approach to reminder/recall that has demonstrated effectiveness in supporting human papillomavirus (HPV) vaccine series completion though has not supported childhood influenza vaccination.[13,14] This may be due to the limited ability for reminder/recall systems to address concerns related to vaccine hesitancy affecting its capacity to positively impact vaccine initiation and blunting its effectiveness.[15] As such, the increased rates of vaccine hesitancy might partially explain the negligible or small impact of reminder/recall systems reported in many recent studies. Given this competing evidence as well as financial considerations, there has been low utilization of the most effective reminder/recall systems by clinics and health care systems.[16]

With advances in technology, other potentially more cost-effective electronic approaches to reminder/recall have been trialed. Email reminders have demonstrated efficacy compared with no intervention.[17] Patient portals, secure Web-based platforms allowing for asynchronous communication between families and providers, offer a promising approach to reminder/recall with increasing usage by health care systems. However, there is currently minimal evidence as to their effectiveness for addressing the vaccine hesitancy determinants. An intervention comparing generic and tailored patient portal reminders did not demonstrate a substantial increase in influenza vaccination rates among adults.[18,19] For children, although portal reminders have not demonstrated effectiveness in increasing first-dose influenza vaccination, they have been associated with an increased receipt of second doses.[20] Although the impact of portal-based interventions may be limited by the large variability in how patients/parents interface with portals,[21] they ultimately do not address many salient determinants of vaccination hesitancy. Specifically, portals have limited ability to effectively address a patient/parent's previous experience with a vaccine, attitudes about prevention, and trust in the health care system and provider.

For provider-level interventions, information systems might support up-to-date vaccination status in patients through clinical decision support. These interventions can take the form as interruptive and non-interruptive reminders of vaccine care gaps by the electronic health record (EHR) to decrease the incidence of missed opportunities to vaccinate. Unfortunately, such automated best practice alerts have not resulted in sustained meaningful increases in influenza vaccine uptake or increased rates of subsequent HPV vaccine doses.[22,23] A randomized controlled multisite trial of incorporation of EHR-delivered provider prompts into routine clinical care did not demonstrate an improvement in adolescent vaccination rates as compared with the standard-of-care control sites.[24] A separate randomized controlled multisite trial found that provider-level EHR-based alerts, as part of a bundle with evidence-based information on addressing vaccination barriers, led to a statistical increase in rates of the first HPV vaccination. However, this did not impact subsequent HPV vaccine doses when compared with controls. When the provider-level alert was combined with automated reminder calls to families with access to educational materials on adolescent vaccination, the rates of vaccine initiation and completion of the HPV vaccine series were significantly increased compared with either intervention alone.[25] Thus, although there may be limited benefit to the use of clinical decision support in isolation, approaches that incorporate provider or patient education to overcome vaccine hesitancy may have more robust impacts on vaccine uptake.

Web-Based Information

Although health care providers are consistently considered a trusted source of vaccine information by families,[26] parents often turn to the Internet as an easily accessible platform for patient-level health information related to vaccines.[27–29] The percentage of US adults who report regular use of the Internet has increased dramatically over the last decade from 79% in 2011 to 93% in 2021.[30] "Vaccine" has become a more common search term over time with a substantial increase in the quantity of information available.[31] When it comes to trusted sources of information on vaccine-safety, online sources governed by physicians groups (eg, the American Academy of Pediatrics) are rated more highly by parents than government or vaccine manufacturer Web sites.[26] Unfortunately, due to a lack of formal monitoring or quality control of user-generated content online, anti-vaccine Web pages are widespread. Platforms such as Twitter, YouTube, Facebook, and Instagram have made it simple for anti-vaccination activists to circulate their messages.[32–35] Moreover, vaccine critical sites with low quality or misleading information are often highly ranked (and presented high in the list of "matching" sites) by Internet search engines due to alignment with search terms focused on risks or safety of vaccination.[31,36] Despite the profusion of anti-vaccine sentiment in certain online communities, the Internet holds the potential for patient/ parent-level interventions to positively impact attitudes around vaccination. A study by McRee and colleagues found that parents searching the Internet for information on the HPV vaccine were associated with higher knowledge and mostly positive attitudes around HPV vaccination for their daughters.[37] O'Leary and colleagues found that sharing reliable Web-based vaccine information with pregnant women increased influenza vaccine uptake.[38] However, identifying reliable information on vaccines can be challenging for both providers and parents.[39] Misinformation related to vaccines is so prevalent that the WHO established a global network of Web sites, the Vaccine Safety Net that identifies reputable resources based on credibility, content, and accessibility.[40] Vaccine Safety Net member Web pages include those from the American Academy of Pediatrics, the Centers for Disease Control and Prevention, and the Institute for Vaccine Safety at Johns Hopkins Bloomberg School of Public Health among over 100 others.[41–43]

When considering provider-level interactions with Web-based information to address determinants of vaccine hesitancy, opportunities exist in the dimensions of advocacy and amplifying factual content. Parents infrequently discuss health information that they find on the Internet or social media with their pediatricians, limiting the opportunities for in-person dispelling of misinformation and provision of high-quality materials to families.[44,45] Thus, it is critical for pediatricians to play an active role in advocating for vaccination on the online platforms most commonly used by patients and families. Unfortunately, such advocacy can open pediatricians to attack from well-organized, coordinated anti-vaccine groups. Organizations such as "Shots Heard Round the World" work to support providers advocating for vaccination on social media that might encounter such an ambush, but challenges still arise.[46] Providers can also demand that online platforms are held accountable for dissemination of disinformation on vaccines due to the negative impact on the health of patients and families. These types of efforts in part motivated Facebook in 2019 to attempt to curtail misinformation through policies that reduced the visibility of anti-vaccine groups, screened vaccine advertisements for accuracy more thoroughly, and attempted to connect users more easily with reputable resources. Such efforts resulted in a decrease in the number of endorsements of anti-vaccine content on Facebook.[47] More work is needed to meet families where they are (online) to disseminate and support positive, consistent vaccine messaging. Please see the article within this volume specifically focused on social media for further discussion on its potential for positively combatting vaccine hesitancy.

Web-based interventions are also a common provider-level approach to vaccine information sharing and have demonstrated a positive impact on attitudes and self-efficacy among clinicians.[48] However, online continuing medical education vaccine interventions do not focus on practical aspects of behavioral/skill training. One study identified Web-based, continuing medical education trainings focused on HPV vaccination and conducted a quality evaluation of the trainings. The evaluation found the trainings provided limited interactivity and completed a limited assessment of providers' knowledge after the training.[49] Furthermore, a content analysis of learning objectives for HPV vaccine online continuing medical education activities found that most objectives focused on low-level learning outcomes (eg, knowledge, comprehension) with very few dedicated to the application of skills. Of the 21 online continuing medical education (CME) activities included in this study, just one of their 68 learning objectives focused on behavior change.[50] Another study that assessed 15 continuing medical education activities related to HPV vaccination found less than 50% of activities included modeling of effective recommendation behaviors or provided clinicians with strategies to address common concerns.[51] With advances in technology, other modalities of training beyond Web-based information sharing might support providers' vaccine recommendation skills by allowing for deliberate practice of skills aligning with educational and behavior change theories.[52]

Mobile Apps

As with the Internet, access to smartphones has increased dramatically over the last decade among US adults from 35% in 2011 to 85% in 2021.[53] A cross-sectional study at an urban pediatric primary care clinic serving a predominantly publicly insured population demonstrated an increase in smartphone ownership from 71% in 2012 to more than 95% in 2017.[8] Thus, mobile apps represent a broadly accessible strategy for patient/parent-level interventions focused on vaccine knowledge and attitudes. Vaccipack, a mobile app using videos, stories, and a discussion forum to support adolescent vaccinations demonstrated high levels of acceptability among adolescents and parents.[54] Another app, Morbiquiz, using quizzes and a leaderboard to support vaccine literacy demonstrated increased knowledge and intention to vaccinate a child for measles, mumps, and rubella.[54,55]

The use of gamified elements (eg, leaderboard, role play, reward systems) is a strategy harnessed by some mobile apps to support user engagement in delivery of health promotion information. Gamification, defined as incorporating gaming elements into non-gaming environments, has demonstrated positive outcomes on cognition and behavior related to vaccination.[56,57] A scoping review on the use of gamification to support vaccine knowledge and attitudes identified seven interventions effective at increasing awareness of vaccine benefits and enhancing motivation for uptake.[58] Five of these interventions were serious games, digital game experiences focused on education rather than entertainment (eg, role play, leaderboard, levels, challenges, and puzzles), and two were quiz-based. These digital interventions demonstrated particular efficacy among children, demonstrating the power of digital technologies may have to deliver positive vaccine messages to children to reduce future vaccine hesitancy.[59] However, gamification is still rarely used to support user engagement in health promotion apps with a recent systematic review noting that just 64 of 1680 health apps included gaming elements. Moreover, apps that incorporated gamification used a variety of embedded behavior change techniques limiting our understanding of what approach is most likely to positively impact patient attitudes toward vaccination.[60]

Other uses for mobile apps include allowing parents to easily track a child's vaccination status to support engagement in up-to-date vaccination status.[61] There are apps that convey specific information to support vaccination among special populations such as pregnant individuals and transplant patients.[62,63] Continued advancements in technology, including artificial intelligence, provide an opportunity to counsel patients and families through chatbots that deliver automated, yet personalized messages. A study in France demonstrated that individuals exposed to a chatbot that delivered adaptive/responsive information on the COVID-19 vaccine resulted in more positive attitudes toward the vaccine and intention to vaccinate when compared with those who received generic information.[64] A continued focus on rigorous assessment of effectiveness of available apps is critical to identifying optimal strategies for positive vaccine messaging, especially given there is no current framework to regulate the development of mobile apps.

Effective interventions for providers on addressing vaccine hesitancy are critical to support consistent, positive vaccine messaging to patients and families.[49] However, as discussed, Web-based information sharing has been limited in terms of focus on practical aspects of behavioral/skill training. As such, mobile apps have been used as a provider-level intervention to support clinicians' communication with families. High-quality vaccine recommendations that have demonstrated effectiveness at supporting vaccine uptake have been successfully incorporated into mobile apps for training.[65,66] One such app, *HPV Vaccine: Same Way, Same Day* developed by the Academic Pediatric Association and the American Academy of Pediatrics in partnership with Kognito, includes simulated role play scenarios during which users counsel a graphical parent hesitant to accept the HPV vaccine for their child.[67] Pediatric residents have described the app as interactive and informative, and usage has resulted in improved knowledge for, attitudes toward, and self-efficacy at counseling on the HPV vaccine.[68,69] Identifying effective technology-based approaches to train clinicians in evidence-based communication is critical to addressing vaccine hesitancy determinants centered on trust for and strength of vaccine recommendations from providers.[70] An important next step for both patient/parent and provider interventions using mobile technology is an assessment of the impact of such interventions on actual vaccination rates, a notable gap in the literature.

Virtual Reality

VR offers unique opportunities to provide patients and families with accurate vaccine information and to combat vaccine hesitancy. VR has been defined as a tool that uses technology to create environments in which individuals can interact with graphical environments and characters in a seemingly realistic way.[71] Among patients and families, VR interventions have demonstrated increased knowledge retention and intention to vaccinate.[72–74] A study by Mottelson and colleagues used a VR consultation with a general practitioner for communicating the benefits of COVID-19 vaccination. Individuals with compatible VR headsets were invited to install the team's experimental application and complete a 10-min virtual consultation. Among the 282 participating adults not previously vaccinated against COVID-19, the prevaccination to postvaccination intentions (score range 1–100) increased significantly and correlated with the vaccination intention 1 week later.[72] The investigators hypothesized that the engaging and immersive aspects of VR supported attitude change among participants. The adaptability of VR might allow for tailoring vaccine information to specific cultural sensitivities and languages. For example, Streuli and colleagues described how they used community-based participatory methods to develop a VR intervention to support vaccine education among a Somali refugee community.[75] In addition to being a helpful resource for information sharing, VR is an effective distraction technique for reducing overall pain and fear during vaccination.[76–79] Despite its potential in addressing patient/parent-level vaccine hesitancy determinants, larger trials are needed to identify how best to incorporate VR education into the flow of routine clinical care. Importantly, as with all technological curricula targeting patients and families, co-creation with the intended audiences will be vital.[75]

When targeting provider-level VR interventions to address determinants of vaccine hesitancy, VR has demonstrated efficacy in training clinicians in high-quality vaccine recommendation behaviors and motivational interviewing competencies.[80] For example, a prior study used a 3D-mounted headset to simulate encounters with a graphical parent hesitant to accept the influenza vaccine for their child. Through provision of real-time feedback after each simulated scenario, clinicians deliberately practiced evidence-based communication strategies relevant to vaccine counseling. Clinicians that underwent the VR training demonstrated a decreased rate of influenza vaccine refusal among their patients compared with a control group that received traditional didactic training.[80] A similar pilot study targeting HPV vaccination and delivering VR content via a screen-based platform demonstrated an 18% increase in HPV vaccine initiation rates among the patients of participating providers when compared with a control group.[81] As with interventions targeting patients/parents, provider focused VR curricula should involve clinicians as key stakeholders during intervention development.[82] Providers have already indicated acceptability for VR-based interventions across the continuum of professional practice from nurses to medical students to pediatric subspecialists.[83–86] With the increasing accessibility and affordability of VR equipment, VR-based interventions supporting practical clinical skill development related to vaccine counseling have strong potential to become more prevalent as optimal implementation strategies are identified.

SUMMARY

Given technology's prevalence in society, we should embrace its potential to effectively impact determinants influencing vaccine hesitancy. However, much work is needed to identify how to optimize technology to address vaccine hesitancy determinants and support vaccine uptake. Researchers using technological interventions to overcome vaccine hesitancy should target high-level outcome metrics such as vaccination rates and measurements of behavior change to identify optimal approaches. Educators should support such work to ensure that technology is applied in consideration of adult-learning theory, a frequent oversight when designing provider trainings. For technology-focused interventions, outcomes related to implementation science should be prioritized alongside effectiveness outcomes to understand their potential for sustainability and scalability.[87] Furthermore, technological interventions should be evaluated through a lens of equity as not all patients and practices have proportionate access to the required resources. To optimize reach and adoption, it is critical that interventions are tested with vulnerable and financially insecure populations as well as individuals that self-identify as technologically challenged to identify potential barriers to widespread dissemination. Ultimately, multipronged interventions that include various strategies to support vaccine uptake such as reminders/recalls, presumptive communication training, and onsite vaccination are needed.[52] Technology may assist such efforts through its ubiquitous presence, potential for automation, and capacity as a platform for innovative training of patients/parents and providers. Pediatric practice requires adaptability, ingenuity, innovation, and resilience to build on our current foundation of promising technology-based strategies to address determinants of vaccine hesitancy and amplify positive vaccine messages.

CLINICS CARE POINTS

- Technological innovations are uniquely positioned to address determinants of vaccine hesitancy and enhance vaccine uptake.
- Patient/parent and provider-level interventions using technology to support vaccine education should align with adult-learning and behavior-change theories.
- Interventions aiming to increase vaccine uptake through technology should include components specifically targeting providers' skills related to addressing vaccine hesitancy.

> • Increased accessibility to the Internet, smartphones, and immersive technologies such as virtual reality provide novel avenues to address determinants of vaccine hesitancy.

DISCLOSURE

None of the authors have any commercial or financial relationships relevant to this article to disclose.

REFERENCES

1. Organization WH. Ten threats to global health in 2019. Available at: https://www.who.int/news-room/spotlight/ten-threats-to-global-health-in-2019. Accessed April 29, 2022.
2. MacDonald NE, Hesitancy SWGoV. Vaccine hesitancy: definition, scope and determinants. Vaccine 2015;33(34):4161–4.
3. Fisher A, Mbaeyi S, Cohn A. Addressing Vaccine Hesitancy in the Age of COVID-19. Acad Pediatr 2021;21(4s):S3–4.
4. Organization WH. Available at: https://cdn.who.int/media/docs/default-source/immunization/besd_progress_report_june2020.pdf?sfvrsn=10a67e75_3. Accessed June, 27 2022.
5. Brewer NT, Chapman GB, Rothman AJ, et al. Increasing Vaccination: Putting Psychological Science Into Action. Psychol Sci Public Interest 2017;18(3):149–207.
6. Mavundza EJ, Iwu-Jaja CJ, Wiyeh AB, et al. A Systematic review of interventions to improve HPV vaccination coverage. Vaccines (Basel) 2021;9(7). https://doi.org/10.3390/vaccines9070687.
7. Pires C. What is the state-of-the-art in clinical trials on vaccine hesitancy 2015-2020? Vaccines (Basel) 2021;9(4). https://doi.org/10.3390/vaccines9040348.
8. Real FJ, DeBlasio D, Rounce C, et al. Opportunities for and Barriers to Using Smartphones for Health Education Among Families at an Urban Primary Care Clinic. Clin Pediatr (Phila) 2018;57(11):1281–5.
9. Berenson AB, Rupp R, Dinehart EE, et al. Achieving high HPV vaccine completion rates in a pediatric clinic population. Hum Vaccin Immunother 2019; 15(7–8):1562–9.
10. Szilagyi PG, Albertin C, Humiston SG, et al. A randomized trial of the effect of centralized reminder/recall on immunizations and preventive care visits for adolescents. Acad Pediatr 2013;13(3):204–13.
11. Jacobson Vann JC, Jacobson RM, Coyne-Beasley T, et al. Patient reminder and recall interventions to improve immunization rates. Cochrane Database Syst Rev 2018;1(1):Cd003941.
12. Kempe A, Saville AW, Albertin C, et al. Centralized reminder/recall to increase influenza vaccination rates: a two-state pragmatic randomized trial. Acad Pediatr 2020;20(3):374–83.
13. Wynn CS, Catallozzi M, Kolff CA, et al. Personalized reminders for immunization using short messaging systems to improve human papillomavirus vaccination series completion: parallel-group randomized trial. JMIR Mhealth Uhealth 2021; 9(12):e26356.
14. Szilagyi PG, Albertin CS, Saville AW, et al. Effect of state immunization information system based reminder/recall for influenza vaccinations: a randomized trial of autodialer, text, and mailed messages. J Pediatr 2020;221:123–31, e4.

15. Kempe A, Stockwell MS, Szilagyi P. The contribution of reminder-recall to vaccine delivery efforts: a narrative review. Acad Pediatr 2021;21(4s):S17–23.
16. O'Leary ST, Crane LA, Wortley P, et al. Adherence to expanded influenza immunization recommendations among primary care providers. J Pediatr 2012;160(3): 480–6.e1.
17. Frascella B, Oradini-Alacreu A, Balzarini F, et al. Effectiveness of email-based reminders to increase vaccine uptake: a systematic review. Vaccine 2020;38(3): 433–43.
18. Szilagyi PG, Albertin C, Casillas A, et al. Effect of patient portal reminders sent by a health care system on influenza vaccination rates: a randomized clinical trial. JAMA Intern Med 2020;180(7):962–70.
19. Szilagyi PG, Albertin CS, Casillas A, et al. Effect of personalized messages sent by a health system's patient portal on influenza vaccination rates: a randomized clinical trial. J Gen Intern Med 2022;37(3):615–23.
20. Lerner C, Albertin C, Casillas A, et al. Patient Portal Reminders for Pediatric Influenza Vaccinations: A Randomized Clinical Trial. Pediatrics 2021;148(2). https://doi.org/10.1542/peds.2020-048413.
21. Szilagyi PG, Valderrama R, Vangala S, et al. Pediatric patient portal use in one health system. J Am Med Inform Assoc 2020;27(3):444–8.
22. Bratic JS, Cunningham RM, Belleza-Bascon B, et al. Longitudinal evaluation of clinical decision support to improve influenza vaccine uptake in an integrated pediatric health care delivery system, Houston, Texas. Appl Clin Inform 2019;10(5): 944–51.
23. Wilkinson TA, Dixon BE, Xiao S, et al. Physician clinical decision support system prompts and administration of subsequent doses of HPV vaccine: A randomized clinical trial. Vaccine 2019;37(31):4414–8.
24. Szilagyi PG, Serwint JR, Humiston SG, et al. Effect of provider prompts on adolescent immunization rates: a randomized trial. Acad Pediatr 2015;15(2):149–57.
25. Fiks AG, Grundmeier RW, Mayne S, et al. Effectiveness of decision support for families, clinicians, or both on HPV vaccine receipt. Pediatrics 2013;131(6): 1114–24.
26. Freed GL, Clark SJ, Butchart AT, et al. Sources and perceived credibility of vaccine-safety information for parents. Pediatrics 2011;127(Suppl 1):S107–12.
27. Jones AM, Omer SB, Bednarczyk RA, et al. Parents' source of vaccine information and impact on vaccine attitudes, beliefs, and nonmedical exemptions. Adv Prev Med 2012;2012:932741.
28. Betsch C, Brewer NT, Brocard P, et al. Opportunities and challenges of Web 2.0 for vaccination decisions. Vaccine 2012;30(25):3727–33. https://doi.org/10.1016/j.vaccine.2012.02.025.
29. RA C, PF A. Use of the internet for health information: United States, 2009. national center for health statistics. Available at: https://www.cdc.gov/nchs/products/databriefs/db66.htm. Accessed April 27, 2022.
30. Center PR. Internet/broadband fact sheet. Available at: https://www.pewresearch.org/internet/fact-sheet/internet-broadband/. Accessed April 27, 2022.
31. Bragazzi NL, Barberis I, Rosselli R, et al. How often people google for vaccination: Qualitative and quantitative insights from a systematic search of the web-based activities using Google Trends. Hum Vaccin Immunother 2017;13(2): 464–9.
32. Johnson NF, Velásquez N, Restrepo NJ, et al. The online competition between pro- and anti-vaccination views. Nature 2020;582(7811):230–3.

33. Broniatowski DA, Jamison AM, Qi S, et al. Weaponized Health Communication: Twitter Bots and Russian Trolls Amplify the Vaccine Debate. Am J Public Health 2018;108(10):1378–84.
34. Tang L, Fujimoto K, Amith MT, et al. "Down the rabbit hole" of vaccine misinformation on youtube: network exposure study. J Med Internet Res 2021;23(1):e23262.
35. Kearney MD, Selvan P, Hauer MK, et al. Characterizing HPV vaccine sentiments and content on instagram. Health Educ Behav 2019;46(2_suppl):37–48.
36. Fu LY, Zook K, Spoehr-Labutta Z, et al. Search engine ranking, quality, and content of web pages that are critical versus noncritical of human papillomavirus vaccine. J Adolesc Health 2016;58(1):33–9.
37. McRee AL, Reiter PL, Brewer NT. Parents' Internet use for information about HPV vaccine. Vaccine 2012;30(25):3757–62.
38. O'Leary ST, Narwaney KJ, Wagner NM, et al. Efficacy of a web-based intervention to increase uptake of maternal vaccines: an RCT. Am J Prev Med 2019;57(4): e125–33.
39. Pineda D, Myers MG. Finding reliable information about vaccines. Pediatrics 2011;127(Suppl 1):S134–7.
40. Organization WH. Available at: https://www.vaccinesafetynet.org. Accessed April 25, 2022.
41. Pediatrics AAo. immunizations. Available at: https://www.aap.org/en/patient-care/ immunizations/. Accessed April 25, 2022.
42. CfDCa Prevention. Vaccine safety. Available at: https://www.cdc.gov/ vaccinesafety/index.html. Accessed April 25, 2022.
43. Health JHBSoP. Institute for vaccine safety. Available at: https://www. vaccinesafety.edu/. Accessed April 25, 2022.
44. Bryan MA, Evans Y, Morishita C, et al. Parental Perceptions of the Internet and Social Media as a Source of Pediatric Health Information. Acad Pediatr 2020; 20(1):31–8. https://doi.org/10.1016/j.acap.2019.09.009.
45. Pehora C, Gajaria N, Stoute M, et al. Are parents getting it right? a survey of parents' internet use for children's health care information. Interact J Med Res 2015; 4(2):e12.
46. Wolynn T, Hermann C. Shots heard round the world: better communication holds the key to increasing vaccine acceptance. Nat Immunol 2021;22(9):1068–70.
47. Gu J, Dor A, Li K, et al. The impact of Facebook's vaccine misinformation policy on user endorsements of vaccine content: An interrupted time series analysis. Vaccine 2022;40(14):2209–14.
48. Pahud B, Elizabeth Williams S, Lee BR, et al. A randomized controlled trial of an online immunization curriculum. Vaccine 2020;38(46):7299–307.
49. Rosen BL, Bishop JM, McDonald SL, et al. Quality of web-based educational interventions for clinicians on human papillomavirus vaccine: content and usability assessment. JMIR Cancer 2018;4(1):e3.
50. Rosen BL, Bishop JM, Anderson R, et al. A content analysis of HPV vaccine online continuing medical education purpose statements and learning objectives. Hum Vaccin Immunother 2019;15(7–8):1508–18.
51. Kornides ML, Garrell JM, Gilkey MB. Content of web-based continuing medical education about HPV vaccination. Vaccine 2017;35(35 Pt B):4510–4.
52. Brewer NT. What works to increase vaccination uptake. Acad Pediatr 2021; 21(4s):S9–16.
53. PEW Research Center. Mobile Fact Sheet. Available at: https://www. pewresearch.org/internet/fact-sheet/mobile/. Accessed April 25, 2022.

54. Teitelman AM, Gregory EF, Jayasinghe J, et al. Vaccipack, a mobile app to promote human papillomavirus vaccine uptake among adolescents aged 11 to 14 years: development and usability study. JMIR Nurs 2020;3(1):e19503.
55. Fadda M, Galimberti E, Fiordelli M, et al. Effectiveness of a smartphone app to increase parents' knowledge and empowerment in the MMR vaccination decision: A randomized controlled trial. Hum Vaccin Immunother 2017;13(11): 2512–21.
56. Rutledge C, Walsh CM, Swinger N, et al. Gamification in action: theoretical and practical considerations for medical educators. Acad Med 2018;93(7):1014–20.
57. Ohannessian R, Yaghobian S, Verger P, et al. A systematic review of serious video games used for vaccination. Vaccine 2016;34(38):4478–83.
58. Montagni I, Mabchour I, Tzourio C. Digital gamification to enhance vaccine knowledge and uptake: scoping review. JMIR Serious Games 2020;8(2):e16983.
59. Wilson K, Atkinson K, Crowcroft N. Teaching children about immunization in a digital age. Hum Vaccin Immunother 2017;13(5):1155–7.
60. Edwards EA, Lumsden J, Rivas C, et al. Gamification for health promotion: systematic review of behaviour change techniques in smartphone apps. BMJ Open 2016;6(10):e012447.
61. Seeber L, Conrad T, Hoppe C, et al. Educating parents about the vaccination status of their children: A user-centered mobile application. Prev Med Rep 2017;5: 241–50.
62. Salmon DA, Limaye RJ, Dudley MZ, et al. MomsTalkShots: An individually tailored educational application for maternal and infant vaccines. Vaccine 2019;37(43): 6478–85.
63. Feldman AG, Moore S, Bull S, et al. A Smartphone App to Increase Immunizations in the Pediatric Solid Organ Transplant Population: Development and Initial Usability Study. JMIR Form Res 2022;6(1):e32273.
64. Altay S, Hacquin A-S, Chevallier C, et al. Information delivered by a chatbot has a positive impact on COVID-19 vaccines attitudes and intentions. J Exp Psychol Appl 2021. https://doi.org/10.1037/xap0000400. No Pagination Specified-No Pagination Specified.
65. Opel DJ, Heritage J, Taylor JA, et al. The architecture of provider-parent vaccine discussions at health supervision visits. Pediatrics 2013;132(6):1037–46.
66. Hofstetter AM, Robinson JD, Lepere K, et al. Clinician-parent discussions about influenza vaccination of children and their association with vaccine acceptance. Vaccine 2017;35(20):2709–15.
67. Interactive K. HPV vaccine: same way, same day. Available at: https://apps.apple.com/us/app/hpv-vaccine-same-way-same-day/id1356847181. Accessed April 28, 2022.
68. Real FJ, Rosen BL, Bishop JM, et al. Usability evaluation of the novel smartphone application, hpv vaccine: same way, same day, among pediatric residents. Acad Pediatr 2021;21(4):742–9.
69. Bishop JM, Real FJ, McDonald SL, et al. Evaluation of HPV vaccine: same way, same day(TM): a pilot study. J Health Commun 2022;1–7. https://doi.org/10.1080/10810730.2021.2021459.
70. Limaye RJ, Opel DJ, Dempsey A, et al. Communicating with vaccine-hesitant parents: a narrative review. Acad Pediatr 2021;21(4s):S24–9.
71. Bracq MS, Michinov E, Jannin P. Virtual reality simulation in nontechnical skills training for healthcare professionals: a systematic review. Simul Healthc 2019; 14(3):188–94.

72. Mottelson A, Vandeweerdt C, Atchapero M, et al. A self-administered virtual reality intervention increases COVID-19 vaccination intention. Vaccine 2021;39(46): 6746–53.
73. Nowak GJ, Evans NJ, Wojdynski BW, et al. Using immersive virtual reality to improve the beliefs and intentions of influenza vaccine avoidant 18-to-49-year-olds: Considerations, effects, and lessons learned. Vaccine 2020;38(5):1225–33.
74. Vandeweerdt C, Luong T, Atchapero M, et al. Virtual reality reduces COVID-19 vaccine hesitancy in the wild. Sci Rep 2022;12(1):4593.
75. Streuli S, Ibrahim N, Mohamed A, et al. Development of a culturally and linguistically sensitive virtual reality educational platform to improve vaccine acceptance within a refugee population: the SHIFA community engagement-public health innovation programme. BMJ Open 2021;11(9):e051184.
76. Chad R, Emaan S, Jillian O. Effect of virtual reality headset for pediatric fear and pain distraction during immunization. Pain Manag 2018;8(3):175–9.
77. Arane K, Behboudi A, Goldman RD. Virtual reality for pain and anxiety management in children. Can Fam Physician 2017;63(12):932–4.
78. Ellerton K, Tharmarajah H, Medres R, et al. The VRIMM study: virtual reality for immunisation pain in young children-protocol for a randomised controlled trial. BMJ Open 2020;10(8):e038354.
79. Kılıç A, Brown A, Aras I, et al. Using virtual technology for fear of medical procedures: a systematic review of the effectiveness of virtual reality-based interventions. Ann Behav Med 2021;55(11):1062–79.
80. Real FJ, DeBlasio D, Beck AF, et al. A virtual reality curriculum for pediatric residents decreases rates of influenza vaccine refusal. Acad Pediatr 2017;17(4): 431–5.
81. Real F, Ollberding N, Meisman A, et al. Impact of a virtual reality curriculum on human papillomavirus vaccination: a pilot trial Am J Prev Med.
82. Real FJ, Meisman A, Rosen BL. Usability matters for virtual reality simulations teaching communication. Med Educ 2020;54(11):1067–8.
83. Zackoff MW, Lin L, Israel K, et al. The future of onboarding: implementation of immersive virtual reality for nursing clinical assessment training. J Nurses Prof Dev 2020;36(4):235–40.
84. Zackoff MW, Real FJ, Cruse B, et al. Medical student perspectives on the use of immersive virtual reality for clinical assessment training. Acad Pediatr 2019;19(7): 849–51.
85. Real FJ, DeBlasio D, Ollberding NJ, et al. Resident perspectives on communication training that utilizes immersive virtual reality. Educ Health (Abingdon) 2017; 30(3):228–31.
86. Real FJ, Hood AM, Davis D, et al. An Immersive virtual reality curriculum for pediatric hematology clinicians on shared decision-making for hydroxyurea in sickle cell anemia. J Pediatr Hematol Oncol 2022;44(3):e799–803.
87. Stockwell MS, Stokley S, Kempe A. Implementing effective vaccination interventions into sustainable 'real world' practice. Acad Pediatr 2021;21(4s):S78–80.

Clinician Communication to Address Vaccine Hesitancy

Douglas J. Opel, MD, MPH

KEYWORDS

- Health communication • Vaccine • Child • Preventive health services

KEY POINTS

- Recent advances in vaccine communication research have yielded a set of effective, evidence-based communication strategies for use by pediatric clinicians to facilitate uptake of childhood vaccines.
- The vaccine communication strategies with the best evidence for increasing uptake of childhood and adolescent vaccines is providing a strong vaccine recommendation and using a presumptive format to initiate the vaccine discussion.
- Current and future vaccine communication research is focused on testing the effectiveness of combination communication strategies as well as identifying and testing strategies that can maintain and build trust with parents.

INTRODUCTION

Although overall vaccination coverage of children in the United States remains high,[1] maintaining current coverage levels is increasingly tenuous. Before the severe acute respiratory syndrome coronavirus 2 (SARS-CoV-2) pandemic, 1 in 5 parents in the United States were hesitant about childhood vaccines,[2] and a small but persistent proportion of parents continued to opt their child out of required school-entry vaccines.[3] This may increase postpandemic because the politicization of the processes to develop and approve a SARS-CoV-2 vaccine[4,5] compromised public trust and confidence in those processes.[6] When also considering the disruptions in childhood vaccine delivery during the SARS-CoV-2 pandemic that have had a negative effect on vaccine coverage,[7] it is clear there is a persistent need to improve and sustain childhood vaccine uptake.

Trust in vaccines and those who develop and recommend them are important factors influencing childhood vaccine uptake.[8,9] It is now well understood, for instance, that pediatric clinicians play an influential role in parent vaccine decision-making. Pediatric clinicians are the most common source of vaccine information for parents,[8] are

Department of Pediatrics, University of Washington School of Medicine, Center for Clinical and Translational Research, Seattle Children's Research Institute, M/S: JMB-6, 1900 Ninth Avenue, Seattle, WA 98101, USA
E-mail address: douglas.opel@seattlechildrens.org

Pediatr Clin N Am 70 (2023) 309–319
https://doi.org/10.1016/j.pcl.2022.11.008
0031-3955/23/© 2022 Elsevier Inc. All rights reserved.

pediatric.theclinics.com

the most trusted source for vaccine-safety information,[10] and can positively influence a parent's vaccine behavior,[11] even among parents with concerns about vaccines.[12]

There are, however, many other important factors influencing childhood vaccine uptake.[13–25] Parent perceptions of the safety of vaccines is one particularly prominent factor.[2,11,26–30] This factor is broadly applicable to all vaccines, as investigators have consistently found a high proportion of parents who have concerns about serious side effects of childhood vaccines[2,28,29] and that there are too many vaccines at once.[2,29] It also is a factor that is especially prominent with specific vaccines, such as measles-mumps-rubella (MMR)[30,31] and SARS-COV-2 vaccines.[32] For instance, despite a wealth of evidence to the contrary,[33] long-term neurodevelopmental side effects have propelled parent safety concerns regarding MMR. Short-term side effects, such as myocarditis, have featured prominently in parent safety concerns regarding SARS-COV-2 vaccines.

Other factors influencing childhood vaccine uptake include parental perceptions of their child's susceptibility to vaccine-preventable diseases[34]; cognitive characteristics of decision-making[35–38]; and social and political factors, such as group norms,[39] social networks,[40,41] and school vaccine mandates.[42] If these personal, social, or political factors yield positive parental attitudes toward vaccination, parental intentions to have their child vaccinated are high, and the child is ultimately vaccinated. However, if these personal, social, or political factors yield negative parental attitudes toward vaccination, such as concerns and doubts about the value or need for vaccines, parental intentions to have their child vaccinated can be low, and the parent may delay or refuse vaccines for their child.

Given the influential role of the pediatric clinician in parent vaccine decision-making, there has been a recent research focus on identifying specific vaccine communication strategies clinicians can use with parents to improve childhood vaccine uptake. Because parents continue to turn to their child's doctor to talk about their concerns about vaccines and view their child's doctor as a trusted source of vaccine information, it is critical that pediatric clinicians have a "communication toolbox" they can utilize in these conversations with parents: a set of effective, evidence-based communication strategies to help facilitate the uptake of childhood vaccines. With recent advances in our understanding of what constitutes effective vaccine communication, clinicians now have more tools than ever in this toolbox.[43,44]

CURRENT EVIDENCE
Strong, high-quality clinician recommendation

A clinician vaccine communication strategy consistently associated with increased uptake of childhood and adolescent vaccines in high-quality studies is providing a vaccine recommendation.[45,46] Important elements of a clinician's vaccine recommendation are the strength and quality of the recommendation. There is higher vaccine receipt among children whose parents receive a very strong clinician vaccine recommendation than those who do not.[47]

Presumptive format

A complementary communication strategy with similarly strong evidence for increased vaccine uptake is a clinician's use of a presumptive format to initiate the vaccine discussion.[19,20,48–50] A presumptive format is one in which the clinician asserts a position regarding vaccines using a closed-ended statement, such as *"Sara is due for several vaccines today"* or *"Well we have to do some shots."*[51] This is in contrast to a participatory format, in which an open-ended question is used to more explicitly invite the parent to voice an opinion, such as *"How do you feel about vaccines today?"*

Clinician use of a presumptive format is associated with increased vaccine uptake, even among parents with negative attitudes about vaccines. For instance, significantly fewer parents with negative vaccine attitudes, as defined as those who scored 50 or more on the validated Parent Attitudes about Childhood Vaccines survey,[52–58] resisted vaccine recommendations when providers used a presumptive (vs participatory) initiation format.[19] In addition, clinicians' repeated use of a presumptive (vs participatory) format with parents with negative vaccine attitudes over several visits, given the longitudinal nature of vaccine administration and discussions, yielded significantly less underimmunization among children.[59] Overall, implementation of the presumptive format in practice has been perceived by clinicians as time saving, easy to use, and a way to promote vaccination as part of routine care.[60]

The presumptive format is likely effective because it leverages choice architecture to achieving a desired goal. Choice architecture refers to how a decision is presented. For instance, a decision can be presented as an opt-in—individuals are required to choose an option—or as an opt-out—the default option occurs when no alternatives are actively chosen.[61] Choice architecture affects the choice made, with most sticking with the default option.[62,63] Use of the presumptive format presents the vaccination decision as opt-out by making vaccination the default option.[38,64] The participatory format is akin to opt-in. The primary driver behind the effectiveness of setting the default option by using an opt-out is likely status quo bias, a cognitive bias inherent to human decision-making that results in an aversion to changing a decision that has already been made.[65,66]

Importantly, utilizing defaults in communication with parents merits careful consideration. Defaults should not be used indiscriminately and are most justifiable where there is a high degree of certainty that an intervention is of low risk and high benefit.[67] Childhood vaccines that are recommended by the Advisory Committee on Immunization Practices fulfill these criteria. Given this justification, as well as the strength of evidence for the presumptive format and a strong clinician vaccine recommendation in improving childhood vaccine uptake, both strategies are now considered as the standard of care in vaccine communication.[68]

By contrast, COVID-19 vaccines authorized for emergency use do not fulfill these criteria.[69] Although these vaccines reached a necessary threshold of evidence to authorize them for emergency use, this threshold needs to be distinguished from the threshold needed to justify using defaults when communicating about these COVID-19 vaccines with parents. This latter threshold involves having high certainty of a vaccine's safety and efficacy resulting from comprehensive study over many decades that has culminated in its full approval by federal oversight agencies and universal recommendation by federal advisory committees. Therefore, although clinicians are encouraged to strongly recommend COVID-19 vaccines authorized for emergency use to parents, use of a presumptive approach to initiate this discussion is less justifiable.

Motivational interviewing

Although a strong recommendation and use of a presumptive format for initiating the vaccine discussion with parents are effective, they are not a panacea. Even with the use of these strategies, a proportion of parents with negative vaccine attitudes will still voice resistance to vaccinating their child.[19] In these situations, additional vaccine communication strategies are needed. One such strategy is motivational interviewing (MI). MI is patient-centered framework for behavior change that helps leverage one's inherent motivation for behaviors.[70–72] There are several MI communication techniques that have been found to be effective even when delivered in a single session.[73,74] Some of these MI techniques and their application to the vaccine encounter are shown in **Fig. 1**.

There is evidence from observational studies to support the use of MI in the vaccination context.[75–79] Evidence from experimental studies, however, have been mixed. One randomized controlled trial (RCT) found no significant effect of a clinician communication strategy based on MI on HPV initiation rates. However, this study was not sufficiently powered to detect a difference in this outcome.[80] Conversely, investigators who conducted a large cluster RCT found a positive effect of MI on HPV initiation and completion rates.[81] In this study, clinicians in intervention practices were trained to use the presumptive format for initiating the HPV vaccine discussion for all parents followed by the use of MI in discussions with parents who voiced resistance to the HPV vaccine. Clinicians in control practices provided usual care. There was a significant increase in HPV vaccine initiation and completion among children of parents who received care in intervention (vs control) practices. The results of a RCT designed to assess the effect of a similar communication strategy on childhood vaccination status by age of 2 years are expected in 2024.[82] A prepost study of this strategy used with parents during health supervision visits of their 2 to 5-year olds resulted in a significant decrease in parent negative attitudes about childhood vaccines.[83]

Other strategies

Other adjunctive clinician vaccine communication strategies with some evidence supporting their effectiveness include (1) pursuing adherence to the recommended vaccines due for the child at a visit despite parent initial resistance and (2) bundling the discussion of all vaccines a child is eligible for at the visit at once. Pursuing adherence

---

Open-ended Questions: helps explore and understand a parent's stance on vaccination
Examples:
- "Tell me more about what you already know?"
- "What might be one good reason to vaccinate your child today?"
- "In your mind, what is the harm if you choose *not* to vaccinate her today?"

Affirmations: improves parent engagement in an open discussion with you by helping them feel supported, appreciated, and understood
Examples:
- "You are a good parent. Your concern shows how much you care about your child's safety."
- "You've always tried to be a good role model for your kids."
- "If you thought the vaccine was safe, you would not hesitate because you want what's best for your daughter."

Reflections: encourages partnerships, deepens rapport, and allows a parent to understand themselves and their motivations on a deeper level; reflections are particularly useful when encountering strong emotion or hesitancy
Examples:
- "You're frightened by what you've read on the Internet."
- "You're really worried and you want to make the best decision."
- "So, it sounds like you're worried about the possibility that the MMR vaccine might cause autism."

Autonomy Support: enhances a parent's sense of control and makes them feel more at ease with the conversation
Examples:
- "That said, this is a decision only you can make."
- "Only you can choose what is best for your child."

Ask Permission to Share: puts parents in a less defensive posture and makes them more receptive to the information you'd like to share
Examples:
- "Could I provide you with some information based on what you just shared?"
- "Would you mind if I shared with you why I think this is such an important vaccine?"
- "I have a different view, may I share it with you?"

Fig. 1. Motivational interviewing skills with examples for the vaccine encounter.

refers to responding immediately to a parent's initial verbal resistance to vaccines with a reiteration of the importance of the recommended vaccines for the child, such as "*He really needs these shots.*"[51] In several observational studies, uptake of vaccines was significantly higher when clinicians pursued their vaccine recommendations (rather than acquiesced) after initial parent verbal resistance.[19,48,84] Bundling the discussion of all vaccines a child is due for at a visit at once is supported by observational work in which investigators found that a concurrent discussion of the influenza vaccine with other vaccines a child was also due for was associated with higher influenza vaccine uptake.[48]

Investigators recently conducted a cluster RCT to test the effect of online educational modules designed to help clinicians integrate several of these communication strategies into their discussions with parents about the HPV vaccine.[85] The clinician communication strategies included were use of a strong recommendation, presumptive format, MI, and bundling. They found a significant reduction in missed opportunities for HPV vaccine initiation in intervention practices compared with control practices.

DISCUSSION AND FUTURE DIRECTIONS

The last decade has yielded several insights into what constitutes effective communication with parents regarding childhood vaccines. Several gaps, however, remain. These gaps are both topical and methodological.

A primary topical gap in our understanding of what constitutes effective clinician vaccine communication is regarding trust. Trust has been associated with vaccine confidence and uptake—trust in the science behind vaccines, trust in the clinicians who administer vaccines, and trust in the institutions that develop, regulate, or recommend vaccines.[86,87] Nonetheless, there is a paucity of evidence regarding how clinicians can nurture and sustain parents' trust in them and the vaccine enterprise.[9] As misinformation and disinformation about vaccines thrives, a key to preserving clinicians as a trustworthy source of vaccine information rests in identifying strategies that effectively address this misinformation and disinformation and help parents maintain trust in their child's pediatric clinician.

Several methodological gaps also need to be addressed. First, we need to target the fence-sitters in research.[88] Parents who have negative attitudes about childhood vaccines or who consider themselves to be hesitant about childhood vaccines are the main population of interest because these are the parents whose vaccine behavior we are most interested in changing. We therefore need to design studies and power trials to detect effects of communication interventions on this population. Too often, interventions that are designed to address negative vaccine attitudes or vaccine hesitancy have been tested among all-comers, rather than the parent subset with negative vaccine attitudes or vaccine hesitancy. This results in little to no understanding of whether the intervention had a positive effect on the population of parents for whom the intervention was primarily intended.

Second, some multicomponent interventions targeting multiple barriers to vaccine uptake simultaneously at the parent-level, clinician- level, and practice-level have been conducted.[89] We need more research. Improving our understanding of what constitutes effective clinician vaccine communication, and subsequently learning how to best incorporate these strategies into practice through implementation science research, is necessary. However, this alone will likely not yield as much of an effect on vaccine uptake as combining clinician communication strategies with additional strategies that target other known factors that influence vaccine uptake. This is as much practical as it is logical: health supervision visits—where most vaccine conversations with parents occur—are already too constrained by time and competing demands. Adjunctive strategies to effective clinician vaccine communication that can occur before and after the clinical encounter are critical to reaching immunization goals.

Finally, there is more to understand about the strategies that we know work. For instance, there is only an early understanding of why the presumptive format is effective at increasing vaccine uptake. Recently, investigators found that a parent's psychological reactance, or propensity to restore their individual autonomy when they perceive others trying to impose their will on them, impacts vaccination intentions.[90] Moreover, this reactance seems to be mediated by the messages they hear from their child's clinician. Presumptive messages to parents with high reactance—messages that they might perceive as limiting or restricting their freedom or choice—negatively impacted vaccination intentions. More research such as this is needed to effectively guide clinicians on how to utilize evidence-based strategies such as the presumptive format.

SUMMARY

There have been incredible recent advances in our understanding of what constitutes effective clinician vaccine communication with parents. Many of these strategies can and should be integrated into clinical practice. More, however, are needed, and if the trajectory of vaccine communication research in coming decade is similar to that of the last, more are sure to come.

CLINICS CARE POINTS

> - High-quality evidence supports the use of a strong vaccine recommendation and a presumptive format to initiate the childhood vaccine discussion with parents, such as *"She is due for several vaccines today."*
> - Other vaccine communication strategies with some evidence supporting their effectiveness include MI, pursuing adherence to the recommended vaccines due for the child at a visit despite parent initial resistance, and bundling the discussion of all vaccines a child is eligible for at the visit at once.

DISCLOSURE

I have no conflicts of interest, whether financial or other.

REFERENCES

1. Hill HA, Yankey D, Elam-Evans LD, et al. Vaccination coverage by age 24 months among children born in 2017 and 2018 - national immunization survey-child, United States, 2018-2020. Mmwr 2021;70(41):1435–40.
2. Santibanez TA, Nguyen KH, Greby SM, et al. Parental vaccine hesitancy and childhood influenza vaccination. Pediatrics 2020;146(6).
3. Seither R, Laury J, Mugerwa-Kasujja A, et al. Vaccination coverage with selected vaccines and exemption rates among children in kindergarten - united states, 2020-21 school year. Mmwr 2022;71(16):561–8.
4. Stolberg S. Trump May Reject Tougher F.D.A. Vaccine standards, calling them 'political. The New York Times 2020.

5. LaFraniere S, Weiland N. White House Blocks New Coronavirus Vaccine Guidelines. The New York Times 2020.

6. Pew Research Center. U.S. Public Now Divided Over Whether To Get COVID-19 Vaccine. September 2020.

7. Santoli JM, Lindley MC, DeSilva MB, et al. Effects of the COVID-19 pandemic on routine pediatric vaccine ordering and administration - United States, 2020. Mmwr 2020;69(19):591–3.

8. Eller NM, Henrikson NB, Opel DJ. Vaccine information sources and parental trust in their child's health care provider. Health Educ Behav 2019;46(3):445–53.

9. Larson HJ, Clarke RM, Jarrett C, et al. Measuring trust in vaccination: a systematic review. Hum Vaccin Immunother 2018;14(7):1599–609.

10. Freed GL, Clark SJ, Butchart AT, et al. Sources and perceived credibility of vaccine-safety information for parents. Pediatrics 2011;127(Suppl 1):S107–12.

11. Gust DA, Darling N, Kennedy A, et al. Parents with doubts about vaccines: which vaccines and reasons why. Pediatrics 2008;122(4):718–25.

12. Smith PJ, Kennedy AM, Wooten K, et al. Association between health care providers' influence on parents who have concerns about vaccine safety and vaccination coverage. Pediatrics 2006;118(5):e1287–92.

13. Ames HM, Glenton C, Lewin S. Parents' and informal caregivers' views and experiences of communication about routine childhood vaccination: a synthesis of qualitative evidence. Cochrane Database Syst Rev 2017;2:CD011787.

14. Mills E, Jadad AR, Ross C, et al. Systematic review of qualitative studies exploring parental beliefs and attitudes toward childhood vaccination identifies common barriers to vaccination. J Clin Epidemiol 2005;58(11):1081–8.

15. Kennedy AM, Brown CJ, Gust DA. Vaccine beliefs of parents who oppose compulsory vaccination. Public Health Rep 2005;120(3):252–8.

16. Taylor JA, Darden PM, Slora E, et al. The influence of provider behavior, parental characteristics, and a public policy initiative on the immunization status of children followed by private pediatricians: a study from Pediatric Research in Office Settings. Pediatrics 1997;99(2):209–15.

17. Kimmel SR, Burns IT, Wolfe RM, et al. Addressing immunization barriers, benefits, and risks. J Fam Pract 2007;56(2 Suppl Vaccines):S61–9.

18. Benin AL, Wisler-Scher DJ, Colson E, et al. Qualitative analysis of mothers' decision-making about vaccines for infants: the importance of trust. Pediatrics 2006;117(5):1532–41.

19. Opel DJ, Heritage J, Taylor JA, et al. The architecture of provider-parent vaccine discussions at health supervision visits. Pediatrics 2013;132(6):1037–46.

20. Opel DJ, Mangione-Smith R, Robinson JD, et al. The influence of provider communication behaviors on parental vaccine acceptance and visit experience. Am J Public Health 2015;105(10):1998–2004.

21. Anderson LM, Wood DL, Sherbourne CD. Maternal acculturation and childhood immunization levels among children in Latino families in Los Angeles. Am J Public Health 1997;87(12):2018–21.

22. Prislin R, Suarez L, Simpson DM, et al. When acculturation hurts: the case of immunization. Social Sci Med (1982) 1998;47(12):1947–56.

23. Gowda C, Dempsey AF. The rise (and fall?) of parental vaccine hesitancy. Hum Vaccin Immunother 2013;9(8):1755–62.

24. MacDonald NE, Hesitancy SWGoV. Vaccine hesitancy: definition, scope and determinants. Vaccine 2015;33(34):4161–4.

25. Handy LK, Maroudi S, Powell M, et al. The impact of access to immunization information on vaccine acceptance in three countries. PLoS One 2017;12(8): e0180759.
26. Bauch CT, Earn DJ. Vaccination and the theory of games. Proc Natl Acad Sci U S A 2004;101(36):13391–4.
27. Evans M, Stoddart H, Condon L, et al. Parents' perspectives on the MMR immunisation: a focus group study. Br J Gen Pract 2001;51(472):904–10.
28. Kempe A, Saville AW, Albertin C, et al. Parental hesitancy about routine childhood and influenza vaccinations: a national survey. Pediatr 2020;146(1).
29. Kennedy A, Lavail K, Nowak G, et al. Confidence about vaccines in the United States: understanding parents' perceptions. Health Aff (Project Hope) 2011; 30(6):1151–9.
30. Ugale JL, Spielvogle H, Spina C, et al. "It's like 1998 again": why parents still refuse and delay vaccines. Glob Pediatr Health 2021;8. 2333794X211042331.
31. Freed GL, Clark SJ, Butchart AT, et al. Parental vaccine safety concerns in 2009. Pediatrics 2010;125(4):654–9.
32. Monitor KFFC-V. Winter Update on Parents' Views (November 8-23, 2021). 2021. Available at: https://www.kff.org/coronavirus-covid-19/dashboard/kff-covid-19-vaccine-monitor-dashboard/. Accessed January 14, 2022.
33. Di Pietrantonj C, Rivetti A, Marchione P, et al. Vaccines for measles, mumps, rubella, and varicella in children. Cochrane Database Syst Rev 2021;11: CD004407.
34. Riddiough MA, Willems JS, Sanders CR, et al. Factors affecting the use of vaccines: considerations for immunization program planners. Public Health Rep 1981;96(6):528–35.
35. Asch DA, Baron J, Hershey JC, et al. Omission bias and pertussis vaccination. Med Decis Making 1994;14(2):118–23.
36. Buttenheim AM, Asch DA. Leveraging behavioral insights to promote vaccine acceptance: one year After disneyland. JAMA Pediatr 2016;170(7):635–6.
37. Meszaros JR, Asch DA, Baron J, et al. Cognitive processes and the decisions of some parents to forego pertussis vaccination for their children. J Clin Epidemiol 1996;49(6):697–703.
38. Opel DJ, Omer SB. Measles, mandates, and making vaccination the default option. JAMA Pediatr 2015;169(4):303–4.
39. Streefland P, Chowdhury AM, Ramos-Jimenez P. Patterns of vaccination acceptance. Social Sci Med (1982) 1999;49(12):1705–16.
40. Brunson EK. The impact of social networks on parents' vaccination decisions. Pediatrics 2013;131(5):e1397–404.
41. Opel DJ, Marcuse EK. Window or mirror: social networks' role in immunization decisions. Pediatrics 2013;131(5):e1619–20.
42. Briss PA, Rodewald LE, Hinman AR, et al. Reviews of evidence regarding interventions to improve vaccination coverage in children, adolescents, and adults. The Task Force on Community Preventive Services. Am J Prev Med 2000;18(1 Suppl):97–140.
43. Limaye RJ, Opel DJ, Dempsey A, et al. Communicating with vaccine-hesitant parents: a narrative review. Acad Pediatr 2021;21(4S):S24–9.
44. Dempsey AF, O'Leary ST. Human papillomavirus vaccination: narrative review of studies on how providers' vaccine communication affects attitudes and uptake. Acad Pediatr 2018;18(2S):S23–7.
45. Smith LE, Amlot R, Weinman J, et al. A systematic review of factors affecting vaccine uptake in young children. Vaccine 2017;35(45):6059–69.

46. Newman PA, Logie CH, Lacombe-Duncan A, et al. Parents' uptake of human papillomavirus vaccines for their children: a systematic review and meta-analysis of observational studies. BMJ Open 2018;8(4):e019206.
47. Dempsey AF, Pyrzanowski J, Lockhart S, et al. Parents' perceptions of provider communication regarding adolescent vaccines. Hum Vaccin Immunother 2016; 12(6):1469–75.
48. Hofstetter AM, Robinson JD, Lepere K, et al. Clinician-parent discussions about influenza vaccination of children and their association with vaccine acceptance. Vaccine 2017;35(20):2709–15.
49. Sturm L, Donahue K, Kasting M, et al. Pediatrician-parent conversations about human papillomavirus vaccination: an analysis of audio recordings. J Adolesc Health 2017;61(2):246–51.
50. Brewer NT, Hall ME, Malo TL, et al. Announcements versus conversations to improve HPV vaccination coverage: a randomized trial. Pediatrics 2017;139(1): e20161764.
51. Opel DJ, Robinson JD, Heritage J, et al. Characterizing providers' immunization communication practices during health supervision visits with vaccine-hesitant parents: a pilot study. Vaccine 2012;30(7):1269–75.
52. Opel DJ, Taylor JA, Zhou C, et al. The relationship between parent attitudes about childhood vaccines survey scores and future child immunization status: a validation study. JAMA Pediatr 2013;167(11):1065–71.
53. Opel DJ, Taylor JA, Mangione-Smith R, et al. Validity and reliability of a survey to identify vaccine-hesitant parents. Vaccine 2011;29(38):6598–605.
54. Opel DJ, Mangione-Smith R, Taylor JA, et al. Development of a survey to identify vaccine-hesitant parents: the parent attitudes about childhood vaccines survey. Hum Vaccin 2011;7(4):419–25.
55. Hofstetter AM, Simon TD, Lepere K, et al. Parental vaccine hesitancy and declination of influenza vaccination among hospitalized children. Hosp Pediatr 2018; 8(10):628–35.
56. Strelitz B, Gritton J, Klein EJ, et al. Parental vaccine hesitancy and acceptance of seasonal influenza vaccine in the pediatric emergency department. Vaccine 2015;33(15):1802–7.
57. Cunningham RM, Minard CG, Guffey D, et al. Prevalence of vaccine hesitancy among expectant mothers in houston, texas. Acad Pediatr 2018;18(2):154–60.
58. Williams SE, Morgan A, Opel D, et al. Screening tool predicts future underimmunization among a pediatric practice in tennessee. Clin Pediatr 2016;55(6): 537–42.
59. Opel DJ, Zhou C, Robinson JD, et al. Impact of childhood vaccine discussion format over time on immunization status. Acad Pediatr 2018;18(4):430–6.
60. Malo TL, Hall ME, Brewer NT, et al. Why is announcement training more effective than conversation training for introducing HPV vaccination? A theory-based investigation. Implementation Sci : IS 2018;13(1):57.
61. Halpern SD, Ubel PA, Asch DA. Harnessing the power of default options to improve health care. N Engl J Med 2007;357(13):1340–4.
62. Ariely D. Predictably irrational. New York, NY: Harper-Collins; 2009.
63. Johnson EJ, Goldstein D. Medicine. Do defaults save lives? Science 2003; 302(5649):1338–9.
64. Renosa MDC, Landicho J, Wachinger J, et al. Nudging toward vaccination: a systematic review. BMJ Glob Health 2021;6(9).
65. Bazerman MH, Moore DA. Judgment in managerial decision-making. New York: Wiley; 2013.

66. Samuelson W, Zeckhauser R. Status quo bias in decision making. J Risk Uncertainty 1988;1(1):7–59.
67. Blumenthal-Barby J, Opel DJ. Nudge or grude? Choice architecture and parental decision-making. Hastings Cent Rep 2018;48(2):33–9.
68. National Center for Immunization and Respiratory Diseases CfDCaP. Talking with Parents about Vaccines for Infants. 2018. Available at: https://www.cdc.gov/vaccines/hcp/conversations/talking-with-parents.html. Accessed Febrary 12, 2022.
69. Opel DJ, Lo B, Peek ME. Addressing mistrust about COVID-19 Vaccines among patients of color. Ann Intern Med 2021;174(5):698–700.
70. Miller WR, Rollnick S. Motivational interviewing: preparing people for change. New York, NY: The Guilford Press; 1991.
71. Rollnick S, Miller WR, Butler CC. Motivational interviewing in health care: helping patients change behavior. New York, NY: The Guilford Press; 2008.
72. Miller WR. Motivational interviewing: research, practice, and puzzles. Addict Behaviors 1996;21(6):835–42.
73. Brand V, Bray K, Macneill S, et al. Impact of single-session motivational interviewing on clinical outcomes following periodontal maintenance therapy. Int J Dental Hyg 2013;11(2):134–41.
74. Hides L, Carroll S, Scott R, et al. Quik fix: a randomized controlled trial of an enhanced brief motivational interviewing intervention for alcohol/cannabis and psychological distress in young people. Psychother Psychosom 2013;82(2):122–4.
75. Gagneur A. Motivational interviewing: a powerful tool to address vaccine hesitancy. Can Commun Dis Rep 2020;46(4):93–7.
76. Lemaitre T, Carrier N, Farrands A, et al. Impact of a vaccination promotion intervention using motivational interview techniques on long-term vaccine coverage: the PromoVac strategy. Hum Vaccin Immunother 2019;15(3):732–9.
77. Gagneur A, Battista MC, Boucher FD, et al. Promoting vaccination in maternity wards horizontal line motivational interview technique reduces hesitancy and enhances intention to vaccinate, results from a multicentre non-controlled pre- and post-intervention RCT-nested study, Quebec, March 2014 to February 2015. Euro Surveill 2019;24(36).
78. Gagneur A, Lemaitre T, Gosselin V, et al. A postpartum vaccination promotion intervention using motivational interviewing techniques improves short-term vaccine coverage: PromoVac study. BMC public health 2018;18(1):811.
79. Glanternik JR, McDonald JC, Yee AH, et al. Evaluation of a vaccine-communication tool for physicians. J Pediatr 2020;224:72–78 e71.
80. Joseph NP, Bernstein J, Pelton S, et al. Brief client-centered motivational and behavioral intervention to promote HPV vaccination in a hard-to-reach population: a pilot randomized controlled trial. Clin Pediatr 2016;55(9):851–9.
81. Dempsey AF, Pyrznawoski J, Lockhart S, et al. Effect of a health care professional communication training intervention on adolescent human papillomavirus vaccination: a cluster randomized clinical trial. JAMA Pediatr 2018;172(5):e180016.
82. Opel DJ, Robinson JD, Spielvogle H, et al. Presumptively Initiating Vaccines and Optimizing Talk with Motivational Interviewing' (PIVOT with MI) trial: a protocol for a cluster randomised controlled trial of a clinician vaccine communication intervention. BMJ open 2020;10(8):e039299.
83. Mical R, Martin-Velez J, Blackstone T, et al. Vaccine hesitancy in rural pediatric primary care. J Pediatr Health Care 2021;35(1):16–22.

84. Shay LA, Baldwin AS, Betts AC, et al. Parent-provider communication of HPV vaccine hesitancy. Pediatrics 2018;141(6).
85. Szilagyi PG, Humiston SG, Stephens-Shields AJ, et al. Effect of training pediatric clinicians in human papillomavirus communication strategies on human papillomavirus vaccination rates: a cluster randomized clinical trial. JAMA Pediatr 2021;175(9):901–10.
86. Sturgis P, Brunton-Smith I, Jackson J. Trust in science, social consensus and vaccine confidence. Nat Hum Behav 2021;5(11):1528–34.
87. Brewer NT, Chapman GB, Rothman AJ, et al. Increasing vaccination: putting psychological science into action. Psychol Sci Public Interest 2017;18(3):149–207.
88. Leask J. Target the fence-sitters. Nature 2011;473(7348):443–5.
89. Rand CM, Tyrrell H, Wallace-Brodeur R, et al. A learning collaborative model to improve human papillomavirus vaccination rates in primary care. Acad Pediatr 2018;18(2S):S46–52.
90. Finkelstein SR, Boland WA, Vallen B, et al. Psychological reactance impacts ratings of pediatrician vaccine-related communication quality, perceived vaccine safety, and vaccination priority among U.S. parents. Hum Vaccin Immunother 2020;16(5):1024–9.

Training Residents and Medical Students to Overcome Parents' Vaccine Hesitancy

Amisha Malhotra, MD, Patricia Whitley-Williams, MD*

KEYWORDS

- Communication • Vaccination • Vaccine hesitancy • Provider communication
- Medical education • Pediatric residency program • Curriculum

KEY POINTS

- Vaccine education should be included in the medical school curriculum.
- A standardized vaccine education curriculum should be included in pediatric residency training programs.
- Knowledge about vaccinology and communication skills can lead to improved discussions with parents and patients with vaccine hesitancy.
- Assessment of knowledge, communication skills, beliefs, and attitudes about vaccines and vaccine hesitancy should be conducted upon matriculation into medical school.
- Medical schools and pediatric residency programs should identify effective strategies to improve the skills of trainees in being able to discuss vaccines with vaccine-hesitant patients and parents.

Evidence-based observations demonstrate that strong provider recommendations increase vaccine confidence.[1] Medical students and residents play an important role in the messaging about childhood and adolescent vaccines to parents. This role becomes increasingly important as the medical student advances to residency and then independent practice as a clinician. Therefore, the rationale for including immunization curriculum in medical school and residency is to ensure that providers have the tools (knowledge and expertise, communication skills, and self-confidence) to be able to conduct well-informed discussions about immunizations with parents.

Division of Pediatric Allergy, Immunology and Infectious Diseases, Department of Pediatrics, Rutgers Robert Wood Johnson Medical School, 1 Robert Wood Johnson Place, New Brunswick, NJ 08901, USA
* Corresponding author.
E-mail address: whitlepn@rwjms.rutgers.edu

Pediatr Clin N Am 70 (2023) 321–327
https://doi.org/10.1016/j.pcl.2022.11.009
0031-3955/23/© 2022 Elsevier Inc. All rights reserved.
pediatric.theclinics.com

THE CURRENT STATUS OF IMMUNIZATION EDUCATION IN MEDICAL SCHOOLS

Very little data are currently available regarding immunization education in medical schools. Vaccine communication training is not currently a standard component of medical school curricula. Studies that have assessed vaccine hesitancy among practicing physicians in the United States, Canada, and Europe report that 22% to 60% are hesitant to routinely recommend certain vaccinations to their patients.[2–5] This hesitancy results in lower immunization rates and vaccine acceptance.[1] An essential step forward in improving immunization rates and vaccine acceptance is by assessing the current education of future physicians about vaccination. In addition to communication training, a decreased ability to understand vaccinology has been reported.

A national survey of Canadian medical, nursing, and pharmacy school students identified important knowledge gaps among most fourth-year students regarding vaccine indications/contraindications, adverse events, safety, and a lack of satisfaction with immunization-related training.[6] In a cross-sectional French study of more than 2000 medical students, more than 50% of the students surveyed felt inadequately prepared to address vaccine hesitancy and/or deal with vaccine refusal, as well as communicate about potential vaccine side effects or discuss the historical impact of vaccination on vaccine-preventable diseases (VPDs) with parents/caregivers.[7] Some of the difficulties in assessing the knowledge level of the students regarding vaccine hesitancy are the lack of standardization of formal medical school training as well as the lack of evaluation of the effectiveness of teaching about vaccine hesitancy.

Upon reviewing the United States Medical Licensure Examination content outline, subject matter related to vaccine safety, vaccinology, as well as communication and interpersonal skills and decision-making abilities is included; however, there is no specific mention of vaccine hesitancy/refusal.[8]

THE CURRENT STATUS OF IMMUNIZATION EDUCATION IN RESIDENCY

Educating all future physicians to confidently recommend vaccination and respond compassionately to vaccine-hesitant parents should be a core component of residency training. Research has shown that teaching communication methods to physicians after residency has been effective at improving physician comfort conversing with vaccine-hesitant parents.[9–12] However, immunization education has not been consistently provided in residency training.[13] A 2014 study found that of 92 pediatric residency programs in the United States, only 41% of programs had formal training in vaccine safety and communication strategies for vaccine-hesitant parents.[13] In another study, members of the Association of Pediatric Program Directors were surveyed as to whether their pediatric residency programs provided formal training in vaccine safety. The response rate was 46.2% of the 199 members, with only 41% of the respondents stating that they included formal vaccine safety training in their residency curriculum. Eighty-one percent of the respondents who did not have vaccine safety training in their residency program curriculum strongly expressed a desire to include such a program. However, there needs to be further research as to what the most effective training methods should be to provide future pediatricians with the skills to effectively communicate with parents about vaccine safety and the benefits of vaccine as well as to effectively address vaccine hesitancy or refusal.[13]

In addition, the historical success of the childhood vaccine program over VPDs may, unfortunately, further complicate resident education in this field. A study by Cordrey and colleagues[14] examined pediatric residents' knowledge of and confidence in recognizing VPDs. Regardless of year of training, most of the residents thought that they were not trained in recognizing many VPDs such as polio, rubella, or diphtheria, and less than a third reported that they could identify measles or mumps. This reflected the high success of the childhood vaccination program in significantly decreasing VPDs to the level that our recent trainees rarely get firsthand exposure to these illnesses. Based on a study by Mergler and colleagues[15] in which 551 providers were surveyed, there was 15% decreased odds in believing in vaccine efficacy compared with a cohort of providers from an earlier 5-year study period. Almost 4% of the providers in the study thought that the risk of vaccination outweighed the benefit. This study suggests that decreased clinical experience with VPDs may be associated with a decreased belief in the safety and benefits from vaccines.

There are several factors that may be contributing to residents' inadequacy when dealing with parental vaccine hesitancy, including:

1. Lack of standardized training about vaccine hesitancy
2. Growing skepticism about vaccine efficacy and benefit
3. Lack of personal or professional experience with VPDs

In addition, the American Board of Pediatrics certifying examination for pediatricians that assesses all core competencies includes topics on routine and catch-up immunization schedules, without mention of vaccine hesitancy in its content outline.[16]

KNOWLEDGE, ATTITUDES, AND BELIEFS REGARDING VACCINATION: ASSESSMENTS AND INTERVENTIONS

It is assumed that our trainees believe in vaccination because they are required to be vaccinated to enter medical school and to work in health care settings. Vaccinations are also required to be done on medical staff of hospitals and ambulatory settings. However, there is a paucity of data published regarding student and resident personal beliefs and attitudes about vaccinations.

General attitudes and beliefs toward vaccination became most apparent during the severe acute respiratory syndrome coronavirus 2 (SARS-CoV-2) epidemic and the introduction of the coronavirus disease 2019 (COVID-19) vaccines to the general public and health care workers. During the COVID-19 pandemic, Polish medical students expressed a higher willingness to get vaccinated against SARS-CoV-2 than the general population. However, the fear of side effects of the SARS-CoV-2 mRNA vaccine decreased vaccine readiness.[17] A similar US study showed that more than 20% of students were COVID vaccine hesitant despite self-perception of elevated risk of exposure to COVID-19 infection. This observation is in contrast to previous studies that show risk perception as a central predictor of protective intentions and preventive health behaviors.[18] Contributing factors to vaccine hesitancy for the COVID-19 vaccine in this group include concerns about serious vaccine side effects and lack of trust in the information received from public health experts.[19] In an anonymous study of residents and fellows at Texas Tech Medical School during the novel COVID-19 pandemic, 96% reported that they wanted vaccination and almost 4% reported that they did not want vaccination.[20] Further assessment of the future health care provider pool needs to be conducted regarding attitudes and beliefs around vaccine self-acceptance and to measure how that may reflect on their messaging to parents. Medical educators should not assume that students and residents adopt the "voice of medicine" about vaccines without addressing their own concerns. However, studies on assessment of knowledge, attitudes, and beliefs regarding vaccinations among trainees have shown that implementation of educational programs using multiple modalities can successfully increase vaccine awareness and improve provider confidence among trainees.[21–23]

An example of such an intervention involved the training of preclinical medical students using a multimodal educational curriculum to improve student knowledge and confidence regarding the human papillomavirus (HPV) vaccine. This educational curriculum was composed of (1) didactic teaching about HPV and the vaccine, (2) a video instruction demonstrating communication skills using both the presumptive method and the C.A.S.E. ([Corroborate, About me, Science, and Explain/advise] is an organized method used in communicating with vaccine hesitant parents.) method, and (3) role-play simulation using both techniques. Results from a presurvey and postsurvey showed an increase in students' awareness of the benefits of the HPV vaccine (27% vs 73%, $P < .01$), the likelihood of recommending the vaccine to both females and males equally, and their comfort level in talking to vaccine-hesitant parents. Finally, students were surveyed about their perceived usefulness of the C.A.S.E method to address HPV vaccine hesitancy in their future clinical encounters. Greater than 90% of students found the C.A.S.E approach useful, not only to talk about vaccine hesitancy but also to discuss other medical concerns.[21]

The CoVER Team (the Collaboration for Vaccine Education and Research) developed a successful online educational curriculum for pediatric and family medicine residents. The development of this curriculum included a needs assessment to measure the perspectives of the program directors and the residents on vaccine education topics as well as a preferred curriculum format. The curriculum consisted of questions on vaccine knowledge as well as vaccine attitudes and hesitancy, using the Parent Attitudes about Childhood Vaccines survey.[24] Results showed that vaccine knowledge was 53% in the preintervention survey and increased in both the intervention and control groups in the postintervention survey. Vaccine hesitancy was more common among family medicine residents than pediatric residents (23% vs 10%). Interestingly, 13% of the residents who completed both the preintervention and postintervention surveys were vaccine hesitant before the intervention. The self-reported vaccine expertise increased in both the control group (from 49% to 56%) and the intervention group (from 46% to 61%). However, the intervention group reported a significantly greater increase in self-confidence in their ability to discuss vaccines with parents compared with the control group ($P < .001$).[24]

Another example of a successful multimodal teaching intervention for entering medical students helped increase provider confidence in discussing influenza vaccines with parents. This intervention included a presurvey and postsurvey, and an interactive session with a librarian, in which students developed and researched their own questions or myths about vaccine hesitancy and participated in peer group discussions followed by a didactic lecture. About half of the students had been vaccinated before entering school. Most of them stated they were vaccinated at the recommendation of family, friends, and/or their primary care physician, indicating the role of societal influence as well as the medical provider in the decision to vaccinate. The postintervention survey showed a significantly improved attitude about influenza vaccination, including a decrease in the number of students who believed that influenza vaccination causes the flu. The postintervention survey also showed that most students (81% compared with 65% on the presurvey) now supported mandatory influenza vaccination for health care workers. There was a significant improvement in perceived comfort in counseling and administration of the vaccination.[25]

Other studies have reported utilization of an objective structured clinical examination (OSCE) station with a standardized patient as an educational tool for a needs assessment in which a resident's communication, interpersonal and counseling skills, as well as effectiveness of discussing vaccination with a live person was assessed. This is an observed encounter, which affords immediate feedback from the standardized patient as well as the faculty observer; this is a suggested educational model for training residents and assessing their ability to manage a patient with vaccine hesitancy.[26] Other suggested educational models include the use of virtual reality curriculum for second- and third-year medical students, which was tested in a pilot study and showed a decrease in influenza vaccine refusal rate.[22]

Even though there are a variety of successful interventions and strategies used to help train medical students and residents to increase provider confidence in discussing vaccine hesitancy/refusal, there is no specific strategy that has been adapted and formalized. However, some of the more successful strategies include interactive group/peer discussions and not just didactic sessions. A review of published papers by the Canadian SAGE Working Group on Vaccine Hesitancy on the effectiveness of strategies to address vaccine hesitancy found no strong evidence to recommend any one intervention.[5] Almost a decade after that paper was published, we are still pursuing effective strategies to address vaccine hesitancy.

FUTURE CONSIDERATIONS AND DIRECTIONS

To help improve understanding and benefit of vaccines among the general public and to decrease vaccine hesitancy/refusal, vaccine education should start well before medical school, as part of healthy lifestyles and disease prevention, and should continue beyond the lifespan of medical training.

Most medical students and residents in the United States are coming from the same communities, as our parents, including those parents who are vaccine hesitant. It is not surprising that these trainees are entering medical school with certain attitudes and beliefs about vaccinations that are reflective of their personal experiences. These trainees have matriculated through our school systems in which there has not been an assessment of the inclusion or absence of vaccine education in school curricula. Perhaps an early introduction to the importance of vaccines and disease prevention should be taught in the schools, which could impact the individual and public beliefs about immunizations. As an example, the Earth Science Literacy Initiative, conducted by the National Science Foundation, is a standardized curriculum being taught in grades K-12, with aims to educate students about the earth and the rapidly changing environment and resource challenges. Perhaps this type of strategy may have an impact on our matriculating medical students' knowledge, beliefs, and attitudes about vaccinations.

In addition to educating the trainees using effective strategies to address vaccine hesitancy and refusal, it is important to note that trainees model behaviors of faculty and mentors who are practicing pediatricians. It is vital that there be ongoing education and assessment of vaccination strategies and communication strategies for dealing with vaccine hesitancy/refusal for the practicing pediatrician and faculty as well. This need was highlighted in a pilot study of pediatric residents in California observing pediatricians discussing vaccinations with their patients. Although almost all of the residents were very familiar how to access the immunization schedule, they reported that observation of pediatricians discussing vaccines with their parents and patients was an important factor in improving their confidence. Most residents (79.1%) reported feeling confident in their ability to discuss vaccines,[27] emphasizing the need for role modeling and direct observation of vaccine communication with vaccine-hesitant parents in the training of medical students and residents.

SUMMARY

Does increase in knowledge, communication skills, and expertise along with the self-confidence in ability to discuss vaccines with parents lead to increased acceptance by parents and address vaccine hesitancy or refusal? Further research is needed to investigate and identify the necessary skills and education tools required for residency training as well as for medical students. Each medical school and residency training program should do a self-assessment of vaccine education in their current curriculum. Medical schools and residency programs should be encouraged to survey their trainee population at matriculation on their preexisting knowledge, attitudes, and beliefs about vaccines. Based on this needs assessment, the curriculum committees can recommend an intervention and then assess the effectiveness of the intervention using strategies discussed in this article and/or novel initiatives developed by the program.

CLINICS CARE POINTS

- There are identified gaps in vaccine knowledge and communication skills among future physicians, making them inadequately prepared to address vaccine hesitancy.
- Strong provider recommendations increase vaccine confidence.
- Ongoing assessment of vaccine knowledge beliefs and communication skills among future physicians in undergraduate and graduate medical education should be conducted.
- Effective vaccine education should be incorporated into the medical school curriculum and pediatric residency training programs to equip future physicians with the knowledge and skills to address vaccine hesitancy.

REFERENCES

1. National Vaccine Advisory Committee. Assessing the state of vaccine confidence in the united states: recommendations from the national vaccine advisory committee. reports and recommendations. Public Health Rep 2015;130:573–95.
2. Bruno DM, Wilson TE, Ghany F, et al. Identifying human papillomavirus vaccination practices among primary care providers of minority, low-income and immigrant patient populations. Vaccine 2014;32:4149–54.
3. Cataldi JR, O'Leary ST, Markowitz LE, et al. Changes in Strength of recommendation and perceived barriers to Human Papillomavirus vaccination: Longitudinal analysis of primary care physicians, 2008-2018. J Pediatr 2021;234:149–53.
4. Verger P, Fressard L, Collange F, et al. Vaccine hesitancy among general practitioners and its determinants during controversies: a national cross-sectional survey in France. EBio Med 2015;2:891–7.
5. Dube E, Gagnon D. MacDonald NE Strategies intended to address vaccine strategies: Review of published reviews. Vaccine 2015;33:4191–203.
6. Pelly LP, Pierrynowski MacDougall DM, Halperin BA, et al. THE VAXED PROJECT: An Assessment of Immunization Education in Canadian Health Professional Programs. BMC Med Educ 2010;10:86.
7. Kerneis S, Jacquet C, Bannay A, et al. Vaccine education of medical students: a nationwide cross-sectional survey. Am J Prev Med 2017;53:E97–104.
8. United States Medical Licensing Examination; USMLE Content Outline. Available at: https://www.usmle.org/sites/default/files/2021-08/USMLE_Content_Outline.pdf.
9. Szilagyi PG, Humiston SG, Stephens-Shields AJ, et al. Effect of training pediatric clinicians in human papillomavirus communication strategies on human papillomavirus vaccination rates: A cluster randomized clinical trial. JAMA Pediatr 2021;175(9):901.

10. Dempsey AF, Pyrzanowski J, Lockhart S, et al. Effect of a health care professional communication training intervention on adolescent human papillomavirus vaccination: a cluster randomized clinical trial. JAMA Pediatr 2018;172(5):e180016.
11. Dempsey AF, O'Leary ST. Human papillomavirus vaccination: Narrative review of studies on how providers' vaccine communication affects attitudes and uptake. Acad Pediatr 2018;18(2):S23–7.
12. Oh NL, Biddell CB, Rhodes BE, et al. Provider communication and HPV vaccine uptake: A meta-analysis and systematic review. Prev Med 2021;148:106554.
13. Williams SE, Swan R. Formal training in vaccine safety to address parental concerns not routinely conducted in US pediatric residency programs. Vaccine 2014; 32:3175–8.
14. Cordrey K, McLaughlin L, Das P, et al. Pediatric resident education and preparedness regarding vaccine-preventable diseases. Clin Pediatr (Phila) 2018; 57(3):327–34.
15. Mergler MJ, Omer SB, Pan WKY, et al. Are recent medical graduates more skeptical of vaccines? Vaccines 2013;1(2):154–6.
16. General Pediatrics Content Outline; In-Training, Certification and Maintenance of Certification Exams; Effective for exams administered September 1, 2017 and after; The American Board of Pediatrics; Available at: https://www.abp.org/ sites/abp/files/gp_contentoutline_2017.pdf
17. Szmyd B, Bartoszek A, Karuga FF, et al. Medical students and SARS-CoV-2 vaccination: attitude and behaviors. Vaccines 2021;9:128.
18. Koski K, Lehto JT, Hakkarainen K. Simulated encounters with vaccine-hesitant parents: arts-based video scenario and a writing exercise. J Med Educ Curric Dev 2018;5. 2382120518790257.
19. Lucia VC, Kelekar A, Afonso NM. COVID-19 vaccine hesitancy among medical students. J Public Health (Oxf) 2021 Sep 22;43(3):445–9.
20. Abohelwa M, Elmassry M, Abdelmalek J, et al. 2019 Novel coronavirus vaccination among post-graduate residents and fellows. J Prim Care Community Health 2021;12:1–5.
21. Schnaith AM, Evans EM, Vogt C, et al. An innovative medical school curriculum to address human papillomavirus vaccine hesitancy. Vaccine 2018;36(26):3830–5.
22. Real FJ, DeBlasio D, Beck AF, et al. A Virtual Reality Curriculum for Pediatric Residents Decreases Rates of Influenza Refusal. Res Pediatr Education 2017;17(4): 431–5.
23. Whitaker JA, Poland CM, Beckman TJ, et al. Immunization education for internal medicine residents: A cluster randomized control trial. Vaccine 2018;36:1823–9.
24. Pahud B, Williams SE, Lee BR, et al. A randomized controlled trial of an online immunization curriculum. Vaccine 2020;38(46):7299–307.
25. Afonso N, Cavanagh M, Swanberg S. 2014. Improvement in attitudes toward influenza vaccination in medical students following an integrated curricular intervention. Vaccine 2014;32:502–6.
26. Wilhite JA, Zabar S, Gillespie C, et al. I don't Trust It": use of a routine OSCE to identify core communication skills required for counseling a vaccine-hesitant patient. J Gen Intern Med 2021;37(9):2330–4.
27. Arora G, Lehman D, Charlu S, et al. Vaccine health beliefs and educational influences among pediatric residents. Vaccine 2019;37(6):857–62.

Social Media and Vaccine Hesitancy
Help Us Move the Needle

Todd Wolynn, MD, MMM[a], Chad Hermann, MA[a],
Beth L. Hoffman, PhD, MPH[b,c],*

KEYWORDS

- Social media • Vaccine hesitancy • Antivaccine movement • Misinformation
- Disinformation • Communication

KEY POINTS

- Although antivaccine sentiment is not new, social media has provided a way for antivaccine activists to organize, grow their numbers, and spread misinformation and disinformation.
- It is not in the financial interest of social media companies to reduce antivaccine misinformation and disinformation on their platforms, so we cannot rely on these companies to eliminate such content.
- Although effective face-to-face communication by pediatric health-care providers is a powerful tool, it is not a scalable solution to address the antivaccine misinformation and disinformation that confront patients and their families on social media.
- It is incumbent on pediatric health-care providers to leverage social media for good and use it to effectively reach patients and their families, who are already on these platforms.

INTRODUCTION

Despite pediatric health-care providers' years of education and training, use of cutting-edge technology, and adoption of ever-improving care algorithms, we are not as impactful as we could be in the promotion and protection and of our patients' health through social media. This marginalization may be due in part to pediatric health-care providers' lack of communication through these platforms, which is where patients and their families increasingly turn for health advice. According to a 2021 survey, more than 75% of adults get some health-related information on social media.[1]

[a] Kids Plus Pediatrics, 4070 Beechwood Boulevard, Pittsburgh, PA 15217, USA; [b] Department of Behavioral and Community Health Sciences, University of Pittsburgh School of Public Health, 130 De Soto Street, Pittsburgh, PA 15261, USA; [c] Center for Social Dynamics and Community Health, University of Pittsburgh School of Public Health, Pittsburgh, PA, USA
* Corresponding author. Department of Behavioral and Community Health Sciences, University of Pittsburgh School of Public Health, 130 De Soto Street, Pittsburgh, PA 15261.
E-mail address: beth.hoffman@pitt.edu
Twitter: @HoffmanBethL (B.L.H.)

Pediatr Clin N Am 70 (2023) 329–341
https://doi.org/10.1016/j.pcl.2022.11.010
0031-3955/23/© 2022 Elsevier Inc. All rights reserved.

If the COVID-19 pandemic had a silver lining, it was the real-world demonstration of human vulnerability in the face of a novel, highly infectious virus. The rapid creation of a safe and effective vaccine for this virus should have resulted in a universal celebration of science, public health, and evidence-based medicine. However, despite attempts by the World Health Organization, Centers for Disease Control and Prevention (CDC), and other health agencies to communicate about the vaccines online, these efforts were no match for the coordination and growth of the modern antivaccine movement and their ability to disseminate misinformation and disinformation powered by social media.[2]

As Dr Paul Offit frequently states, "Vaccines are a victim of their own success."[3] Although children in the United States have earned a significant degree of safety from infectious diseases due to robust vaccine research and development, rigorous review and approval, careful guidelines and policies, surveillance and monitoring, as well as successful distribution and vaccination platform,[4] problems with vaccine uptake persist.

Lack of vaccine uptake can be explained by the 5 As: Access, Affordability, Awareness, Acceptance, and Activation.[5] Although Access and Affordability remain a problem, particularly for historically marginalized communities, the last 3 As—Awareness, Acceptance, and Activation—are also key barriers. Billions have been spent globally on vaccine research and development,[6] but substantially less has been invested in better understanding and addressing lack of vaccine acceptance (ie, vaccine hesitancy).[7] This is particularly concerning as we are in a golden age of antivaccine misinformation and disinformation,[1,8] with the rapid spread of this content fueled by social media.[9] Behavior change is hard even when humans know right from wrong[10]; it is exponentially harder when caregivers fear vaccinating their children thanks to a steady stream of exposure to antivaccine content on social media.

It is important to clarify some terms: *antivaccine* refers to people in complete opposition to one or more vaccines; *vaccine-hesitant* refers to a continuum of people skeptical or concerned about vaccines who have good-faith questions. It is understandable that, given the exposure to so much vaccine misinformation and disinformation, many caregivers will have concerns about vaccines.

Antivaccine tactics are sophisticated and nuanced, and social media allows narrow targeting of messages intended to create fear based on an individual's beliefs, values, and situation.[11] A 2020 study that used social network analysis to examine how nearly 100 million people who expressed views about vaccines on Facebook interacted with each other found that those who espouse antivaccine views are well connected to people who express vaccine hesitancy but people who espouse provaccine views are mostly only connected to others who express provaccine views. In other words, people on Facebook who post provaccine content mostly interact with like-minded people, whereas those who post antivaccine content often reach out to those who express hesitancy. They accomplish this, in part, by tailoring their messages to specific audiences with narratives tied to safety, conspiracies, and alternative medicine.[12] This study also found that provaccine narratives, in contrast, are relatively uniform and not well tailored to address different vaccine-related concerns.[12] These findings explain how antivaccine misinformation and disinformation can travel so quickly on social media and exert such a powerful effect on the vaccine hesitant.

It is critical to engage those who are vaccine hesitant with respect, attention, active listening, empathy, and evidence-based answers. Although engaging face-to-face with vaccine-hesitant caregivers is important, it is also essential to engage them virtually. Social media platforms are inexpensive, easy to master, and able to reach tens (or hundreds) of thousands more people daily than can possibly be seen in an office. It is particularly important for individual practitioners and practices to use these platforms because they can build on the trust they establish in the examination room.

In this article, we will first review the ways in which the antivaccine movement has leveraged social media to expand their considerable influence, as well as why social media companies have failed to reduce antivaccine misinformation and disinformation. We will then review barriers to adoption of social media-based communication by pediatric health-care providers, and close with action-oriented items to increase the adoption of this powerful tool by providers and health systems.

Like a Fish to Water: the Antivaccine Movement Goes Social

Organized efforts to oppose vaccination campaigns have grown simultaneously with vaccinology. Andrew Wakefield is frequently identified for taking the antivaccine movement into prime-time in the late 1990s, using fraudulent research to advance his claims.[13] His more than 15 seconds of fame exposed his fraudulent research and conflicts of interest and ultimately cost him his medical license but not before damaging confidence in the MMR vaccine.[13]

Before social media, antivaccine groups were loosely organized and aligned with both the political right (on concepts of freedom and liberty) and the political left (on concepts of trust and purity). Their resources were limited but they maintained a devoted following, fueled in part by celebrities such as Charlie Sheen and Jenny McCarthy.

Social media changed the game, allowing those across the political aisles to unite, grow their ranks, secure funding, and organize.[14] The antivaccine movement's use of social media since the early 2010s positioned them to deny facts, control trends, and impact caregivers and politicians alike. The COVID-19 pandemic, coupled with the increase of political radicalism on the right (also fueled by social media), created an opportunity for the burgeoning antivaccine movement.[15] During the pandemic, social media promotion of misinformation and disinformation expanded to multiple antiscience stances such as antimask, antishutdown, antimandates, and anticontact tracing, all aligning with and adding fuel to the antivaccine stance. Furthermore, prior research has found that Russian social media trolls (people who post intentionally provocative or offensive messages to get attention or cause trouble) and bots (automated software that help spread particular messages) push antivaccine rhetoric and purposely try to foment distrust in public health agencies in the United States, all while supporting pro-nationalism efforts.[16]

The antivaccine movement has also mastered the art of highly coordinated attacks on vaccine advocates. In 2017 Kids Plus Pediatrics, an independent practice in Pittsburgh, Pennsylvania, received tens of thousands of antivaccine comments and threats from around the globe on a video promoting the human papillomavirus vaccine.[17] A 2020 event designed to promote vaccination on Twitter—#DoctorsSpeakUp—was overtaken by a coordinated antivaccine presence.[18] An analysis of Twitter messages (ie, tweets) with this hashtag on the day of the event found that almost 80% were antivaccine, with most antivaccine tweets being one of 6 prewritten tweets disseminated by antivaccine activists before the event. The ability of antivaccine activists to coopt this event was due not only to their swift ability to organize but also the relatively small numbers of pediatric health-care providers and other vaccine advocates who use social media to promote vaccination.

Social Media Exploitation of Human Behavior Vulnerabilities

The ability of antivaccine rhetoric to spread on social media is due in large part to social media algorithms exploiting human behavior vulnerabilities to promote the spread of false information. In the days of television and print media, a single phrase reflected how to get viewers and reader attention: "If it bleeds, it leads!" In the age of social media, that mantra has become: "If it scares, it shares."[2] A 2018 study found that false information diffuses faster than truth on Twitter,[19] and one can imagine a post claiming "vaccines cause cancer" will spread much more quickly on social media than a factual, and thus not sensational, post proclaiming "550 million doses of COVID vaccines have been administered in the U.S. with outstanding safety and effectiveness."

The software engineers who program social media algorithms do not work in a vacuum. They are supported by myriad experts in social science, linguistics, risk, and decision-making who understand how to leverage the innate human response to detect and respond to perceived threats.[19] Humans are hard-wired to respond to fear, so seeing a frightening message, video, or post triggers an urge to "like" or "share" content quickly, often before reading the full post and almost always before validating the accuracy of the content.[20] Although it is easy to blame trolls and bots for the problem of the rapid spread of sensational and divisive content, it is far too often "ordinary" users who amplify this propaganda.[20]

The algorithms leverage another innate factor: humans are social creatures. Most people not only seek out connectedness with others but strive to be liked. Research has found that cognitive biases related to social interaction function differently online compared with offline.[21] For example, people may be more attuned to cues indicating in-group versus out-group status online,[22] meaning when people see their social networks sharing misinformation or disinformation, they may be more likely to accept it than if they encountered it offline. Research has also found that when we post/contribute/share content, we are encouraged to repeat this action because we receive our version of a reward—an endorphin spike—in the form of a like, share, and/or follow.[23] In other words, "click-bait" is real, and it works!

These human behavioral vulnerabilities can be manipulated and monetized.[24] To social media platforms, each click equates to money in the form of advertisement revenue and billions of posts, likes, and shares translate to hundreds of billions of dollars of revenue annually.[25] A recent analysis by the Center for Countering Digital Hate estimates that the advertisement revenue connected to antivaccine content alone amounts to more than US$1 billion a year, likely explaining why social media companies continue to turn a blind eye to the harm this content causes.[26] Although they repeatedly make gestures and promises to police themselves, it is simply not in their financial interest to reduce misinformation or disinformation. Furthermore, social media companies are not liable for false information on their platforms due to Section 230 of the Communications Decency Act, which states that no "provider or an interactive computer service shall be treated as the publisher...of any information provided by another."[27] In other words, although the author of a particular social media post can be sued for defamation, the social media platform itself cannot be. Because of extensive lobbying by social media companies, repeal of Section 230 is unlikely.[27]

Barriers to Adoption of Social Media: the Caged Pediatrician

In 2008, only 10% of Americans reported having a social media profile. By 2021, that number increased to 79%.[28] Internet health-related inquiries are common; Google Health Vice President David Feinberg, MD, claims there are more than 1 billion health queries daily.[29] Recognizing the power of social media as a behavior change tool,[30] in 2020 US corporations spent US$40 billion on social media advertisements.[31] Despite this power, pediatric health-care providers have yet to understand, invest in, and use this vast resource for behavior change.[32]

Although systems-level social media (eg, Kaiser Health System) can be created, the innate trust based on authentic personal-professional relationships carries more social media cachet and connectedness. Families want reliable, trusted, expert guidance when making decisions about their children. Health-care professionals are the most trusted profession in the United States, and pediatricians are near the top of the list[33]—likely due to the longitudinal relationships, often decades long, that pediatric providers have with families. This trust is precious and powerful.

In considering why relatively few pediatric health-care providers to date have successfully leveraged this trust with social media-based communication, it should be noted that pediatric providers face barriers related to training, perpetuation of health communication fallacies, lack of system-level support, fear of negative repercussions, and concerns about equity.

Training: Pheochromocytoma Versus Facebook

Health-care professional training programs, including medical schools, frequently highlight their adaptations to our changing world to reflect advances in areas such as epigenetics, technological advances, and the application of big data.[34] However, these newer topics still compete with ageless issues such as: *"A 42 year old male presents with headache, palpitations and diaphoresis… need another hint… headaches…What is the diagnosis?"*

If you have not yet diagnosed pheochromocytoma, take note, as you will likely see this on at least 2 to 3 key examinations you will take for licensure. Although we have nothing against familiarity with neuroendocrine tumors, we are perplexed about why we are continually testing medical professionals on a rare tumor occurring in 2 to 8 per 1,000,000 people, which they will likely never see in practice. Even without specific suspicion for pheochromocytoma, these persistent symptoms would almost certainly result in workup, which would lead to a correct diagnosis. There are much more common medical topics pediatric providers encounter that should receive much more time, for example, sleep, breastfeeding, social determinants of health, and health equity.

Now imagine the potential for better care if health-care professionals received more training on communication, for example, how to be a better communicator; where to communicate: in person and online; what to do when faced with hesitancy or distrust; and sources of communication that most influences patients and families. Communication expertise is a critical resource that must become a part of all health-care fields. Communication training should start in health-care professional schools, be expanded upon in advanced training or residency, and practiced, supported, and updated throughout health-care careers.

The Two Health-Care Communication Fallacies

Pediatric providers have been traditionally been trained to believe 2 health-care communication fallacies: (1) you can only give advice to patients inside the 4 walls of an examination room and (2) you will be believed (**Fig. 1**).

Unfortunately, the US health-care system pressures providers to minimize good communication in service to charting rapidly and generating more RVUs.[35] Providers are already overwhelmed having to see 20 or more patients per day, and in each annual visit there are far too many important topics to cover everything your families want and need to know.[36] As of June 2022, only about 30% of 5 to 11-year olds have completed their primary series of safe and effective COVID-19 vaccinations.[37] If a pediatric provider wants to be effective in reaching and influencing families at a population-based level in 2022 and beyond, then that provider must be where caregivers live and learn every day—on social media.

The Two Pediatric Communication Fallacies

1. You can only give advice to patients inside the four walls of an exam room.

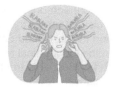

2. You'll be believed.

Fig. 1. The 2 health-care communication fallacies.

Lack of Support

In addition to the health-care communication fallacies (see **Fig. 1**), several institutional barriers inhibit pediatric providers' ability to use social media. The first relates to concerns about how social media pushes information to users. Pulling information, as its name suggests, involves using online resources to "pull" the information you desire, such as using a search engine to look up a movie review, restaurant rating, or weather forecast. In contrast, a "push" occurs when social media applications deliver information to you, in a timeline or newsfeed, based on your history, your likes, and your preferences on the platform. When you "pull" information, you get what you want to see. When social media apps "push" information, you get what they want you to see. This feature of social media contributes to providers being unsure about its use for professional communication.

Our experience suggests the primary reason health-care providers were slow to adapt to, and still often avoid using, social media professionally is because of a lack of financial compensation and professional recognition. There is currently a generational disconnect: decision-making authority (ie, senior physicians or administrators) are typically Generation X (born 1965–1980) or older, and less familiar and/or comfortable with the use of social media.[38] In contrast, Generation Y and Z providers grew up immersed in technology and find using social media second nature but many of them are not empowered to make business decisions about its use in daily practice.

Thus, despite the ability of social media to reach and impact thousands of patients and families each week, very few providers are incentivized or encouraged to post on social media.[39] As a result, the time that providers spend engaging on social media is often at the expense of other activities such as time with loved ones.[39]

Regarding professional recognition, social media engagement is rarely valued by tenure or promotion committees for those in academic spaces.[39] Furthermore, practitioners with authority tend to be highly risk-adverse, and so overinflate or misinterpret liability and communication risks (such as HIPAA violations) commonly associated with social media use. It is not uncommon for health-care organizations to have strict regulations around employee use of social media in a professional capacity, or to have privacy controls or content blockers on work devices that prevent providers from accessing social media sites.[39]

Fear of Negative Repercussions

Senior physicians or administrators may also fear online criticism. However, this fear is misplaced, as such criticism can occur whether one has a social media profile or not. In fact, a social media profile allows providers to better see and respond to what is being said about them and provides an avenue for online support from the families in their practice. Additionally, many pediatric health-care providers fear being on the receiving end of an online attack if they post provaccine content.[22] Although it is true that the antivaccine movement uses tactics of social media harassment to scare trusted and knowledgeable social media vaccine advocates,[40] it should be noted that there are an increasing number of resources available to help. One such resource, the nonprofit group Shots Heard Round the World, was formed in the aftermath of the 2017 antivaccine attack on Kids Plus Pediatrics.[41] This organization provides resources to help vaccine advocates to prevent, defend against, and recover from coordinated online antivaccine attacks, and has effectively come to the aid of pediatricians attacked on social media for advocating vaccines—most famously in the case of Dr Nicole Baldwin.[42] Shots Heard Round the World also provides a support network to vaccine advocates leveraging social media to promote vaccination.[41]

EQUITY CONCERNS

A final concern related to professional social media use is equity. Because social media use requires WiFi or hard-wired connectivity, there are justifiable concerns that it does not reach all people well. This concern has been documented in both rural and underserved urban areas. As a result, lower socioeconomic-status communities struggle with access to this virtual information exchange.[43] Additionally, older, lower technology and cheaper devices and phone carrier plans can also exacerbate inequities regarding access and end-user experience. As a result, it is essential that social media outreach not replace in-person communication but rather be used as a tool to enhance existing on-the-ground outreach.

Social Pediatrics: Trust and Evidence-Based Recommendations via Social Media

Given these barriers, it is understandable that even pediatric health-care providers who understand the value of using social media to reach their families may struggle to adopt this powerful tool. In this section, we review action-oriented items to help providers become ADEPT at using social media (**Table 1**). First, with so many social media platforms out there, providers may wonder which platform to start using. We recommend starting with a single platform, and having that platform be the one with the greatest participation by caregivers of children of the practice. It may be helpful to conduct a brief survey of caregivers or informally assess this during clinic visits. Related to this, remember that the primary audience for your posts is families of the practice. They trust you and can help amplify your message.

When it comes to creating or posting content, keep it interesting and keep the primary audience in mind. It may be helpful to remember frequently asked questions in the examination room and then create or share content to address these topics. The content should be regularly posted and engaging but does not need to be original. Rather, providers can quickly *amplify* trusted voices such as the American Academy of Pediatrics (AAP), AAP's HealthyChildren.org, and the CDC. Sharing content from these sources on a provider or practice-level account serves as a trusted endorsement of this content and the institutions that provide it (see **Table 1**). This can be done in conjunction with *directing* patients and families to resources, either from your practice or these trusted voices (see **Table 1**). If providers find they have time to *post* new content, this can be a great opportunity to *tag* colleagues, thereby easily sharing the content created with other providers and practices. Finally, when engaging with caregivers and/or patients who ask questions or comment on posts, make sure to *engage* with empathy (see **Table 1**).

Table 1
How pediatricians can become adept at using social media to promote vaccination

Tasks	Description	Examples
Amplify trusted voices	Repost (eg, share, retweet) content from trusted health sources such as the CDC, AAP, or local health department	• Share a post by the CDC about influenza vaccines for children • Share a post by the AAP addressing misinformation about COVID-19 vaccines for children
Direct patients to resources	Post information about local vaccine clinics or clinic-related events	• Share a post from the health department about a COVID-19 vaccine clinic • Post a copy of an infographic you have hanging in your waiting room about an influenza vaccine clinic
Engage with empathy	When patients and caregivers ask good-faith questions about vaccines, respond with empathy and compassion	• Respond to a caregiver expressing confusion about Moderna vs Pfizer COVID-19 vaccines for young children by acknowledging that it can be difficult to wade through all of the information online
Post new content	Be creative! Post engaging content that addresses issues you think is most pertinent to your patients and caregivers	• Create a TikTok video to a catchy song informing adolescents about the HPV vaccine • Create an Instagram post addressing FAQs about COVID-19 boosters for children
Tag colleagues	Use each platform's tagging features to easily share the content you create with other pediatric health-care providers	• Tag the HPV Roundtable in a picture you post as part of a tweet encouraging HPV vaccines for boys and girls • Tag individual providers in your practice in a clinic Instagram post about COVID-19 vaccine availability

In the absence of a trusted pediatric provider on social media, caregivers or patients may turn to nonreputable sources offering advice, which could be unintentional misinformation or purposeful disinformation. Thus, whether creating new content or sharing content from reputable sources, a primary goal should be providing evidence-based information before people are exposed to misinformation or disinformation. Research has shown that when people receive factual information before hearing misinformation or disinformation—also known as "prebunking"—it acts as a kind of inoculation, making them less susceptible to the misinformation or disinformation.[44] Social media can also be used as a "fact-check," to address concerns generated by previous exposure to vaccine misinformation or disinformation. As with in-person communication, social media messages must express empathy without reinforcing the disinformation. Similar to the Announce, Inquire, Mirror, Secure method for in-office vaccine conversations,[45] social media posts should first state the facts about the recommended vaccination, next dispel the misinformation or disinformation, and finally conclude with further information or support for the evidence-based vaccine recommendation.[2]

A Call to Action

It is incumbent on medical schools, pediatric training programs, other health training programs, professional medical organizations, and health systems to adapt to the realities of social media. Although face-to-face opportunities are powerful, they are not a scalable solution to the dilemma facing pediatric providers and practices. The multiple competing priorities facing providers makes reaching families on social media with factual pediatric health-care recommendations imperative. Social media provides a significant source of information—and misinformation and disinformation—for families and caregivers. Not maintaining a pediatric provider (or at least practice-level) presence on at least one key social media platform opens the door for parents and caregivers to consume advice from a range of questionable and even nefarious sources. Social media can be used for good but doing so requires a commitment on the part of both providers and health-care systems. With effective use of social media, the precious and trusted longitudinal relationships pediatric providers create with families in the examination room can be both enhanced and fortified; educational content will be welcomed by the many families who enjoy trusted longitudinal relationships with the practice providers. The barrier to entry is low, and social media is an inexpensive, efficient, effective tool to engage, educate, and affect health change at a population level. Social media use offers pediatric providers and practices the ability to reach and affect thousands of patients and families each week, with desired and needed pediatric health-care recommendations. In 2022 and beyond, it is paramount that a pediatric provider (or at least at the practice-level) has a social media presence on at least one social media platform to help effectively counter the contagion of online misinformation and disinformation. We invite you to review the following resources, and then join us in harnessing social media for good.

Resources

CDC Social Media Tools, CDC Social Media Tools: https://www.cdc.gov/socialmedia/tools/index.html.

Shots Heard Round the World: https://shotsheard.org/

Social Media for Doctors, Social Media for Doctors: Taking Professional and Patient Engagement to the Next Level:https://www.aafp.org/pubs/fpm/issues/2020/0100/p19.html.

Social Media –, Social Media – How to harness its power and avoid its traps:https://www.contemporarypediatrics.com/view/social-media-how-to-harness-its-power-and-avoid-its-traps.

CLINICS CARE POINTS

Pitfalls
- Clinical office visits are increasingly packed with multiple competing priorities, making addressing vaccine hesitancy in the office extremely challenging.
- Social media is being used by antivaccine advocates to spread misinformation and disinformation.

Pearls
- Social media is inexpensive to learn and use, relatively easy to master, and its impact can be significantly scaled in a relatively short timeframe to create significant change.
- Health-care leaders/decision-makers must educate themselves so that they might harness this powerful communication and behavior-change tool.
- Health-care social media must become normalized and be incorporated in training so that pediatric health-care providers can use it to positively influence patients and families.

- Most younger providers are intimately familiar with the use of social media. Health-care systems and practices should support and nurture these users and leverage their experience and knowledge professionally.

DISCLOSURE

T. Wolynn has received funding from Merck Corporation and Sanofi Pasteur Inc. for conference travel, lodging, and consulting but not during the time this article was written. T. Wolynn is also cofounder of "Shots Heard Round the World." C. Hermann is cofounder of "Shots Heard Round the World." B.L. Hoffman has no conflicts of interest, real or perceived, to disclose.

ACKNOWLEDGMENTS

The authors would like to thank Riley Wolynn for her assistance with article preparation.

REFERENCES

1. Neely S, Eldredge C, Sanders R. Health Information Seeking Behaviors on Social Media During the COVID-19 Pandemic Among American Social Networking Site Users: Survey Study. J Med Internet Res 2021;23(6):e29802. https//www.jmir.org/2021/6/e29802.
2. Wolynn T, Hermann C. Shots heard round the world: better communication holds the key to increasing vaccine acceptance. Nat Immunol 2021;22(9):1068–70.
3. Hoffman J. How anti-vaccine sentiment took hold in the United States - the New York times. The New York Times. Available at: https://www.nytimes.com/2019/09/23/health/anti-vaccination-movement-us.html. Published September 23, 2019. Accessed June 2, 2022.
4. Vos T, Kyu HH, Pinho C, et al. Global and National Burden of Diseases and Injuries Among Children and Adolescents Between 1990 and 2013: Findings From the Global Burden of Disease 2013 Study. JAMA Pediatr 2016;170(3):267–87.
5. Thomson A, Robinson K, Vallée-Tourangeau G. The 5As: A practical taxonomy for the determinants of vaccine uptake. Vaccine 2016;34(8):1018–24.
6. Kiszewski AE, Cleary EG, Jackson MJ, et al. NIH funding for vaccine readiness before the COVID-19 pandemic. Vaccine 2021;39(17):2458.
7. Reber S, Kosar C. Vaccine hesitancy is an old problem in need of new ideas. Milbank Memorial Fund. Available at: https://www.milbank.org/2022/02/vaccine-hesitancy-is-an-old-problem-in-need-of-new-ideas/. Published June 1, 2022. Accessed June 3, 2022.
8. Puri N, Coomes EA, Haghbayan H, et al. Social media and vaccine hesitancy: new updates for the era of COVID-19 and globalized infectious diseases. Hum Vaccin Immunother 2020;16(11):2586.
9. Stein RA. The golden age of anti-vaccine conspiracies. Germs 2017;7(4):168.
10. Bouton ME. Why behavior change is difficult to sustain. Prev Med (Baltim) 2014;0:29.
11. Brewer NT, Chapman GB, Rothman AJ, et al. Increasing vaccination: putting psychological science into action. Psychol Sci Public Interest 2018;18(3):149–207.
12. Johnson NF, Velásquez N, Restrepo NJ, et al. The online competition between pro- and anti-vaccination views. Nature 2020;582(7811):230–3.

13. Deer B. How the case against the MMR vaccine was fixed. BMJ 2011;342:c5347.
14. Susarla A. Big tech has a vaccine misinformation problem – here's what a social media expert recommends. The Conversation. Available at: https://theconversation.com/big-tech-has-a-vaccine-misinformation-problem-heres-what-a-social-media-expert-recommends-164987. Published July 29, 2021. Accessed June 2, 2022.
15. Lagman JDN. Vaccine nationalism: a predicament in ending the COVID-19 pandemic. J Public Health (Bangkok) 2021;43(2):e375–6.
16. Broniatowski DA, Jamison AM, Qi S, et al. Weaponized health communication: twitter bots and russian trolls amplify the vaccine debate. Am J Public Health 2018;108(10):e1–7.
17. Hoffman BL, Felter EM, Chu K-H, et al. It's not all about autism: the emerging landscape of anti-vaccination sentiment on Facebook. Vaccine 2019;37(16):2216–23.
18. Hoffman BL, Colditz JB, Shensa A, et al. #DoctorsSpeakUp: Lessons learned from a pro-vaccine Twitter event. Vaccine 2021;39(19):2684–91.
19. McCall JM. Media spread fear, Americans listen | The Hill. The Hill. Available at: https://thehill.com/opinion/technology/556160-media-spread-fear-americans-listen/. Published May 30, 2021. Accessed June 2, 2022.
20. DiResta R. It's Not Misinformation. It's Amplified Propaganda. - The Atlantic. The Atlantic. Available at: https://www.theatlantic.com/ideas/archive/2021/10/disinformation-propaganda-amplification-ampliganda/620334/. Published October 9, 2021. Accessed June 2, 2022.
21. Youngblood M. Extremist ideology as a complex contagion: the spread of far-right radicalization in the United States between 2005 and 2017. Humanit Soc Sci Commun 2020;7(1):1–10.
22. Abrams Z. The anatomy of a misinformation attack. American Psychological Association. Available at: https://www.apa.org/monitor/2022/06/news-misinformation-attack. Published June 1, 2022. Accessed June 9, 2022.
23. The Social Dilemma: Social Media and Your Mental Health. McLean | Harvard Medical School Affiliate. Available at: https://www.mcleanhospital.org/essential/it-or-not-social-medias-affecting-your-mental-health. Published January 21, 2022. Accessed June 2, 2022.
24. Hao K. How Facebook and Google fund global misinformation | MIT Technology Review. MIT Technology Review. Available at: https://www.technologyreview.com/2021/11/20/1039076/facebook-google-disinformation-clickbait/. Published November 20, 2021. Accessed June 2, 2022.
25. Beveridge C. 56 Important Social Media Advertising Stats for 2022. Hootsuite. Available at: https://blog.hootsuite.com/social-media-advertising-stats/. Published February 24, 2022. Accessed June 2, 2022.
26. The anti-vaxx industry how big tech powers and profits from vaccine misinformation. Cent Countering Digit Hate 2020. https://doi.org/10.1177/0963721417718261.
27. Jurecic Q. The politics of Section 230 reform: Learning from FOSTA's mistakes. Brookings. Available at: https://www.brookings.edu/research/the-politics-of-section-230-reform-learning-from-fostas-mistakes/. Published March 1, 2022. Accessed June 4, 2022.
28. Surprising Social Media Statistics - The 2022 Edition - BroadbandSearch. Broadband Search. Available at: https://www.broadbandsearch.net/blog/social-media-facts-statistics. Published 2022. Accessed June 2, 2022.

29. Murphy M. Dr Google will see you now: Search giant wants to cash in on your medical queries. Telegraph. Available at: https://www.telegraph.co.uk/technology/2019/03/10/google-sifting-one-billion-health-questions-day/. Published March 10, 2019. Accessed June 2, 2022.
30. Sanchez-Paramo C, Legovini A. Using social media to change norms and behaviors at scale. World Bank Blogs. Available at: https://blogs.worldbank.org/voices/using-social-media-change-norms-and-behaviors-scale. Published January 12, 2021. Accessed June 3, 2022.
31. Social network advertising spending in the United States from 2016 to 2022. Statista. Available at: https://www.statista.com/statistics/736971/social-media-ad-spend-usa/. Published February 23, 2022. Accessed June 2, 2022.
32. Hoffman BL, Boness CL, Chu K-H, et al. COVID-19 Vaccine Hesitancy, Acceptance, and Promotion Among Healthcare Workers: A Mixed-Methods Analysis. J Community Health June 2022. https://doi.org/10.1007/S10900-022-01095-3.
33. Bailey M. A new study reveals moms' most trusted sources of information. Marketing to moms coalition and current lifestyle marketing. (Non-peer reviewed research report). Available at: https://www.cdc.gov/healthcommunication/pdf/thisjustin/tji_18_200912.pdf. Published September 18, 2008. Accessed June 2, 2022.
34. Buja LM. Medical education today: All that glitters is not gold. BMC Med Educ 2019;19(1):1–11.
35. Himmelstein DU, Woolhandler S, Gaffney A. The US's broken healthcare system is at the root of vaccine hesitancy - the BMJ. BMJ Opinion. Available at: https://blogs.bmj.com/bmj/2021/09/10/the-uss-broken-healthcare-system-is-at-the-root-of-vaccine-hesitancy/. Published September 10, 2021. Accessed June 2, 2022.
36. Weber DO. How Many Patients Can a Primary Care Physician Treat? American Association for Physician Leadership. Available at: https://www.physicianleaders.org/news/how-many-patients-can-primary-care-physician-treat. Published February 11, 2019. Accessed June 2, 2022.
37. Children and COVID-19 Vaccination Trends. American Academy of Pediatrics. Available at: https://www.aap.org/en/pages/2019-novel-coronavirus-covid-19-infections/children-and-covid-19-vaccination-trends/. Published May 25, 2022. Accessed June 2, 2022.
38. Auxier B, Anderson M. Social media use in 2021 | pew research center. Pew Research Center. Available at: https://www.pewresearch.org/internet/2021/04/07/social-media-use-in-2021/. Published April 7, 2021. Accessed June 2, 2022.
39. Panahi S, Watson J, Partridge H. Social media and physicians: Exploring the benefits and challenges. Health Inform J 2016;22(2):99–112.
40. Vogels E. The State of Online Harassment. Pew Research Center. Available at: https://www.pewresearch.org/internet/2021/01/13/the-state-of-online-harassment/. Published January 13, 2021. Accessed June 9, 2022.
41. Shots Heard Round The World. Available at: https://www.shotsheard.com/. Published 2019. Accessed May 25, 2020.
42. Glynn E. Vaccines: TikTok video of Cincinnati doctor Nicole Baldwin goes viral. Cincinnati Enquirer. Available at: https://www.cincinnati.com/story/news/2020/01/17/pediatrician-refuse-back-down-amid-anti-vaccine-backlash/4499119002/. Published January 17, 2020. Accessed June 4, 2022.
43. Vogels EA. Digital divide persists even as Americans with lower incomes make gains in tech adoption. Pew Research Center. Available at: https://www.pewresearch.org/fact-tank/2021/06/22/digital-divide-persists-even-as-americans-

with-lower-incomes-make-gains-in-tech-adoption/. Published June 22, 2021. Accessed June 2, 2022.

44. Roozenbeek J, van der Linden S, Nygren T. Prebunking interventions based on "inoculation" theory can reduce susceptibility to misinformation across cultures. Harv Kennedy Sch Misinformation Rev 2020;1(2). https://doi.org/10.37016//MR-2020-008.

45. Attwell K, Dube E, Gagneur A, et al. Vaccine acceptance: Science, policy, and practice in a 'post-fact' world. Vaccine 2019;37(5):677–82.

Optimizing Your Pediatric Office for Vaccine Confidence

Patricia Stinchfield, RN, MS, CPNP-PC*, Joseph Kurland, MPH, CIC,
Pamela Gigi Chawla, MD, MHA

KEYWORDS

- Vaccine confidence • Pediatric office • Provider trust • No missed opportunities

KEY POINTS

- Pediatric offices must promote trust at each visit and by every staff member to gain vaccine confidence.
- There should be no missed opportunities to vaccinate by treating every visit as a vaccine visit.
- Principles from patient safety, quality improvement, and effective communication can help optimize vaccine confidence.
- A vaccination infrastructure is an imperative lead by a vaccine champion who specializes in staying abreast of vaccine policy changes.

DISCUSSION

Practice Proven Strategies to Increase Vaccine Confidence in the Pediatric Clinic–Office Considerations

Building a culture of safety and trust in the pediatric office

Vaccination in a pediatric office setting is a complex operational process that requires clinicians, staff, parents, and patients to be on the same page. As Stokley[1] noted in the executive summary for improving vaccination coverage issue in Academic Pediatrics, "Multifaceted interventions that include feedback reports, prompts, and education may be the most promising at increasing vaccination coverage." Freed and collegues[2] found parents trust their children's doctors and other health care staff the most (76% endorsed "a lot of trust") for vaccine information over other sources. When all works well, children are vaccinated completely on the recommended immunization schedule, parents are well-informed promoting vaccine confidence, and clinicians are smoothly providing "one of the most successful and cost-effective, life-saving public health tools for preventing disease and death" according to Offit and

---

[a] Children's Minnesota, 2525 Chicago Avenue, Minneapolis, MN 55404, USA
* Corresponding author.
E-mail address: Stinc021@umn.edu

Pediatr Clin N Am 70 (2023) 343–357
https://doi.org/10.1016/j.pcl.2022.11.011   **pediatric.theclinics.com**
0031-3955/23/© 2023 Elsevier Inc. All rights reserved.

DeStefano.[3] Using principles from patient safety, infection control, effective communication, and trust-building literature can support effective vaccination practices. An office culture is built by effective leadership, accountability, dedication to continual quality improvement, and open communication. Staff emulate leaders they trust who role model respectful, knowledgeable patient education. Staff can speak up and feel supported in having vaccine conversations at every step of the clinic operation. Authentic leaders build trust in their pediatric office when they provide psychological safety for staff to speak up, and staff feel that they are a mutually respected part of the team. Staff in turn can have respectful, open communications with parents seeking information, which promotes vaccine confidence.

Patient safety principles as applied to vaccination
Patient safety in health care has long focused on hospital inpatient improvements such as steps to reduce central line–associated bloodstream infections or medication administration errors. Often the Swiss Cheese model[4] is used to describe ways to prevent such errors (**Fig. 1**). Pediatric office settings that administer vaccines can use this same model to take a systems approach in reducing errors in vaccine administration, which helps promote parental confidence in vaccination.

Clinics care points
Steps in an office setting to promote patient safety[4] during vaccination would include the following:

- Develop an office culture that is consistent with the organization's vaccine goals.
- Promote age-eligible vaccines for all children and adolescents.
- Have clear, current, complete evidence-based policies that support safe vaccination.
- Work as an interdisciplinary team, with every team member recognizing the high importance of vaccination.
- Define and maintain clear roles and responsibilities.
- Provide optimal clinician/staff training and continuing education on new vaccines.
- Agree to reduce missed opportunities to vaccinate by making every visit a vaccine visit.
- Emphasize proper administration techniques and pain control, including distractions.

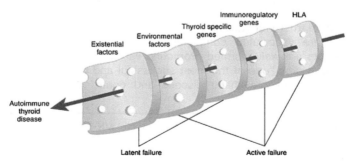

Fig. 1. Swiss Cheese Error Model. (Weetman A, P: The Immunopathogenesis of Chronic Autoimmune Thyroiditis One Century after Hashimoto. Eur Thyroid J 2012;1:243-250. doi: 10.1159/000343834.)

- Develop clear parental roles in holding/comforting children during vaccination.
- Establish whose role it is to inform of when to return to stay on schedule.

Shah and colleagues[5] noted that immunization pain is the "most common cause of iatrogenic pain of childhood."[6] The Children's Comfort Promise was developed at Children's Minnesota as a bundle of interventions used to reduce needle pain. The core aspects include the use of numbing at the injection site, sucrose or breastfeeding during vaccination for infants, and positioning and distraction for all ages. Clinics can learn more about the importance of reducing needle pain by viewing The Children's Comfort Promise video[7] (YouTube link The Children's Minnesota Comfort Promise). Because needle phobia can be a significant barrier for children and adults to getting vaccinated,[8] clinics should have a consultant to work with such as a psychologist or child life specialist who can help patients with desensitization, deep breathing techniques, and other interventions to decrease the anxiety that vaccinations cause in some people.

Transparency in evaluating every vaccine error for improvements
Because the vaccination schedule and process are complex with numerous considerations including right age, right number of doses, right interval from last dose, right technique, right co-administration with other vaccines or other biologicals, and so forth, the possibility for vaccination errors is high. The most common reports to the Centers for Disease Control and Prevention's (CDC) Vaccine Adverse Events Reporting System (VAERS)[9] regarding COVID-19 vaccine, for example, are vaccine administration errors. When errors occur, it reduces the family's confidence with vaccination and the pediatric office, potentially leading to incomplete vaccination. The following steps should happen when a vaccination error occurs:

- Follow a preestablished system to transparently report errors within your office setting to leaders
- Determine if the error meets one of the required VAERS table of reporting events following vaccination (**Fig. 2** shows the VAERS table of reportable events following vaccination).
- Report the error to VAERS either online, by email at info@vaers.org, or by phone at 1-800-822-7967.
- Transparently communicate the error to the family including what to expect by way of potential side effects.
- Consult with vaccine specialists or the manufacturer on whether to repeat the dose and when.
- Document the error for further vaccine committee review and discussion for quality improvements.
- Use quality improvement best practices for system improvements to prevent future errors including measuring error frequency, providing staff feedback, and implementing system improvements as needed.[10]

Pediatric office infrastructure
Clinics should be properly equipped and ready to administer vaccines to patients when the patients are ready to be vaccinated. Staff are key to a clinic functioning smoothly.[11] Educated, trained, and confident staff who can speak to questions around immunization products and procedures can increase the likelihood that patients will stick to the CDC vaccine schedule. For patients who raise concerns for adverse event risks, clinicians can put into context the importance of immunizations against the history of the diseases they prevent. However, once the decision to be vaccinated is made, having products ready to administer is important. Delays and requiring a patient

VAERS Table of Reportable Events Following Vaccination*	
Vaccine/Toxoid	**Event and interval** from vaccination**
Tetanus in any combination; DTaP, DTP, DTP-Hib, DT, Td, TT, Tdap, DTaP-IPV, DTaP-IPV/Hib, DTaP-HepB-IPV	A. Anaphylaxis or anaphylactic shock (7 days) B. Brachial neuritis (28 days) C. Shoulder Injury Related to Vaccine Administration (7 days) D. Vasovagal syncope (7 days) E. Any acute complications or sequelae (including death) of above events (interval - not applicable) F. Events described in manufacturer's package insert as contraindications to additional doses of vaccine (interval - see package insert)
Pertussis in any combination; DTaP, DTP, DTP-Hib, Tdap, DTaP-IPV, DTaP-IPV/Hib, DTaP-HepB-IPV	A. Anaphylaxis or anaphylactic shock (7 days) B. Encephalopathy or encephalitis (7 days) C. Shoulder Injury Related to Vaccine Administration (7 days) D. Vasovagal syncope (7 days) E. Any acute complications or sequelae (including death) of above events (interval - not applicable) F. Events described in manufacturer's package insert as contraindications to additional doses of vaccine (interval - see package insert)
Measles, mumps and rubella in any combination; MMR, MMRV, MM	A. Anaphylaxis or anaphylactic shock (7 days) B. Encephalopathy or encephalitis (15 days) C. Shoulder Injury Related to Vaccine Administration (7 days) D. Vasovagal syncope (7 days) E. Any acute complications or sequelae (including death) of above events (interval - not applicable) F. Events described in manufacturer's package insert as contraindications to additional doses of vaccine (interval - see package insert)
Rubella in any combination; MMR, MMRV	A. Chronic arthritis (42 days) B. Any acute complications or sequelae (including death) of above event (interval - not applicable) C. Events described in manufacturer's package insert as contraindications to additional doses of vaccine (interval - see package insert)
Measles in any combination; MMR, MMRV, MM	A. Thrombocytopenic purpura (7-30 days) B. Vaccine-strain measles viral infection in an immunodeficient recipient o Vaccine-strain virus identified (interval - not applicable) o If strain determination is not done or if laboratory testing is inconclusive (12 months) C. Any acute complications or sequelae (including

Fig. 2. VAERS table of reportable events following vaccination*.

to reschedule an appointment may result in decreased patient satisfaction, an increased chance of a missed opportunity if they do not return, and an unnecessary prolonged exposure risk for vaccine preventable disease, particularly during outbreaks.[12] To be ready, an effective clinic requires a diverse set of equipment and supplies including the following.

Make every visit a vaccine visit

This phrase is an important one in helping pediatric offices build their vaccination culture. If every staff person is dedicated to this concept, it will reduce missed opportunities to vaccinate. Clinics, large or small, should have a system of measuring their

Equipment	Supplies	Policies

Vaccine storage units
Stand-alone
  fridge/freezer
  units
Data logging
  temperature
  monitoring devices
  with battery backup;
  ideally those with
  audible alerts for
  in-clinic staff.
Battery backup for
  storage units in
  sites that don't
  have backup
  generators.[13]
	Alcohol wipes
	Patient skin and
	  aseptic vial access
	Needles, sizes
	  appropriate
	  for patients
	  seen in clinic
	Vaccine products;
	  clearly labeled
	Bandages
	Comfort measure
	  supplies for
	  distraction
		Documentation process
		  providing record of dose,
		  product, vaccine
		  expiration date, lot number,
		  route, location, and
		  date administered
		Automated
		  Scan patient ID and
		    product packaging
		  Automatically links to
		    patient record in
		    electronic health record
		Manual
		  Process to document
		    doses accurately
		    and effectively
		  Verification steps to
		    minimize errors

Educational resources
  including Vaccine
  Information Statements
  (VIS) as required by
  federal law[14]
Visual reminders
  posted in clinics
  such as the immunization
  schedule, infographics,
  and clear message
  posters as created
  by several sources[15–18]
	—	Appointment scheduling
		Sign up for reminder recall
		  system (phone, fax, email, portal)
		Ensure next vaccine visit is
		  arranged before patient
		  departs clinic

successes.[19] Rand and Humiston[20] describe key factors necessary in building a clinic system that operationalizes this concept: these factors include (1) assessment and feedback, which may boost motivation; (2) interventions to decrease missed opportunities during visits such as previsit planning or huddles that inform provider prompts or standing orders; and (3) communication training to manage vaccine hesitancy. Another important practice-based strategy is reminder/recall messages to parents about needed vaccinations. Reminder/recall remains one of the most effective measures to increase vaccination rates and should be a priority for clinics to implement. Staff must look at the child's vaccination record, not only at well-child visits, but every visit, to determine if they are up-to-date for age on their vaccinations; this works best when one role is consistently responsible for determining if vaccines are needed, prompting a clinician decision. Specifically, Jaca and colleagues[21] found "moderate certainty evidence that the following interventions probably improve vaccination coverage: patient education, patient tracking using community health workers, and …provider prompts." Maximizing the electronic medical record to deliver prompts of overdue vaccination is another example of a tool that can help reduce missed opportunities to vaccinate.[22] In their helpful framework, Proctor and colleagues[23] adapt a general implementation strategy to vaccination strategies highlighting the importance of clearly defining *who* will implement *what* specific action. Continuous quality improvement (CQI) principles are critical for clinics to use to ensure their practice is implementing the best practices that meet the needs of their patients and families.

Using a CQI model such as Plan-Do-Study-Act[24] can help clinics optimize their best practices (**Fig. 3**).

Professionally trained staff build confidence by sensitively administering vaccines while being attentive to pain, families' time, and language needs
Vaccine hesitancy has been a growing issue for the past decade or more. Although those refusing vaccines are in a minority, confidence in vaccine safety, need, and schedules has waned. Numerous polls have indicated that, despite social media influences casting doubt, the source most parents and patients trust with their immunization decisions is their clinician. The relationship and confidence patients have with their medical care team plays a critical role in keeping patients on the CDC-recommended schedule and protected against disease.[25]

Opposition to vaccines presents a constantly evolving challenge for clinicians and medical staff. Trained staff who are well versed in vaccine practices are knowledgeable about common vaccine adverse events, and paying attention to social media may best be able to address the variety of questions and current concerns raised by parents and patients.

Beyond knowledgeable, well-supplied staff, the clinic environment works to instill confidence and trust in patients. Facilities in good repair with organized, clean, and calm environments promote safety for patients and staff.[26] Clinic rooms with calming decor or art that can help distract children and adolescents work to the benefit of the

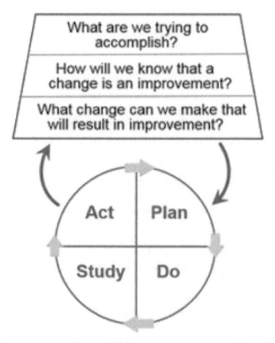

Fig. 3. Model for improvement. The model for improvement provides a framework for rapid testing and change leading to improvement. This model consists of 2 parts: addressing 3 fundamental questions and then engaging in tests of change using the Plan-Do-Study-Act cycle. (*From* Langley G.J., Nolan, K.M., Nolan, T.W, Norman, C.L., & Provost L.P. (2009). The Improvement Guide: A practical approach to enhancing organizational performance (2nd Ed.). San Francisco: Jossey-Bass. P.24.)

vaccinator. Clean and organized vaccine stations and medication prep spaces can decrease error potential and minimize the risk for product contamination.[27]

Clinics or health systems may choose to designate a dedicated team member as "vaccine champion." Formalizing vaccine operations oversight into a dedicated position in the organization called "Vaccine Specialist" clarifies roles, responsibilities, and accountabilities. This individual can serve as an immunization subject matter expert with training and education based on the Clinical Vaccinology Course through the National Foundation for Infectious Diseases.[28] The person in this role is tasked with understanding details around special vaccine product considerations and advising clinical teams in the organization and community medical partners accordingly. The Vaccine Specialist monitors reports about adverse events, new products, recalls, and updated practice guidelines and, in turn, keeps the organization informed. Such an individual can provide staff training and updates, monitor social media for themes, and help draft talking points for clinical staff. The person in the Vaccine Specialist role can serve as a member of an interdisciplinary clinic system vaccine committee who meet regularly to review vaccination rates, new Advisory Committee on Immunization Practices recommendations, new products, and oversight of storage and handling, among other considerations. The established vaccine committee and Vaccine Specialist role can quickly pivot as needed (eg, with the COVID pandemic) to discuss alternative implementation approaches to vaccinating a wider audience, such as with mobile vaccine clinics, drive-through clinics, or mass clinics.

The Vaccine Specialist can identify vulnerabilities and areas for improvement for the clinic and enact change including the following:

- Federal Vaccine for Children product storage and handling requirements and the need for an organization-wide temperature monitoring system with data loggers
- Streamline immunization documentation and reporting to the state immunization registry in partnership with health information management and information technology
- Readiness for emergency response with battery backup and vaccine repacking supplies to move to an alternate site in line with CDC's Storage and Handling Toolkit[29]
- Improve patient outreach and follow-up through appointment reminders and recall services to boost vaccine series compliance and correct intervals
- Standardize vaccine administration equipment, in particular syringe and needle options with common safety device products across the organization to minimize needlestick injuries in staff who float between sites
- Encourage honest, timely, and nonpunitive reporting of vaccine administration errors so appropriate patient follow-up and care can be provided

In addition, to engage staff in achieving high vaccination rates, specialists can co-lead a quality improvement project such as one to reduce missed opportunities or review refusal documentation. Areas for staff to measure and improve include influenza vaccine uptake in patients and staff, child and teen vaccine rates, or measuring missed opportunities by age. Involving all staff will increase the culture of vaccination readiness. Follow national and state measurement guides and compare your clinic, select a disease-specific initiative such as human papillomavirus vaccine to focus on for a year, and create a quarterly improvement award for staff recognition.

Equal and equitable access for all patients, families, and communities promotes trust
Clinics play an important role, along with public health, in ensuring vaccination rates remain high in all communities. Of the necessary fundamentals to ensure high

protective immunization rates, intentionality must be dedicated to the balance between "equal" and "equitable" approaches. Although both are critical, an "equal" approach (communities all get the same intervention such a single site mass immunization clinic day) alone could result in vaccination outcomes that increase health disparities; and an approach that is equitable alone (communities provided with what they need such as a mobile clinic to their local community center) may not achieve a background rate high enough to approach community herd immunity.

In surveys and focus groups of Hispanic, Somali, and Ethiopian adolescents and their parents, Greenfield and colleagues[30] described barriers that pediatric offices should reduce, which included

"...limited awareness of, and misperceptions regarding, recommended adolescent vaccines and vaccine preventable diseases, lack of health care professional (HCP) recommendations for vaccination and inability to access health information in native languages...Lack of knowledge of adolescent vaccination recommendations was the main reason given by parents that their adolescents had not been vaccinated. Most parents identified doctors as a trusted source of health information and reported that they would vaccinate their teens if their doctor recommended it." The study recommended that "HCP's may benefit from guidance on communicating with ethnic populations to support meaningful dialogue with families about the risks and benefits of adolescent vaccines."

Understanding the populations the pediatric office serves and building a staff that reflects the patient population

Clinicians must understand the pediatric population the clinic serves, should be serving, and strategically is planning to serve. Standard demographics such as race and ethnic groups, language, or insurance plotted against vaccination rates are readily acquirable from most electronic medical records or from local or state health departments. However, this alone does not raise the unique cultural needs of the patient and family. Clinics must also attend to transportation needs, religious beliefs, newcomer status to the country or community, their experience with anti-vaccine messaging, and the community's past relationship with the clinic on aspects of care, such as preventative health. Most importantly, building a workforce of staff and clinicians who look like and speak the primary language of the patients will improve trust and will ensure equitable outcomes. According to Ma, "Race/ethnicity concordance significantly increases the likelihood of seeking preventative care for Hispanic, African-American, and Asian patients relative to White patients."[31]

Scheduling tips to maximize vaccine conversations

For families to consent for vaccination, they must have time to both ask questions and have their questions answered. It is helpful for families to have a firm grasp on the anticipated vaccine schedule ahead of any vaccine visit, so that they can come prepared with questions.[32] From the first newborn visits in the clinic onward, it is important to set the expectation for families that vaccinations will occur in upcoming visits and engage in any questions that they (or their extended family) may have ahead of time. If there are specific vaccinations that subsets of patients have concerns about, consider an individualized patient approach to address concerns, such as extending the length of the visit or an additional visit. Ideally, a Vaccine Specialist in an OB-GYN office could begin to fill the parents' information needs early and throughout the pregnancy visits regarding maternal and infant vaccination, much like lactation specialists assist mothers with breastfeeding.

Using all modalities to enhance parental trust—vaccine-only visits, after-hours/ weekend availability, drive-up clinics, mass clinics, and partnerships outside of clinics such as school
Although the clinic framework for vaccination safety is built on standardization and best practices, successful outcomes in vaccination rates are built on accessibility, ease, and trust. Arbitrary limitations in vaccination offerings to specific types of clinic visits, specific hours of the clinic day, or even within the clinic itself may create barriers to access for vaccinations. By understanding your patients' and families' demographics and needs, models for vaccination efforts may be considered to specifically address equitable care. Within the clinic, easy access to vaccine-only visits, order sets for administration, and after-hours vaccinations would be a consideration that may allow busy families to remain up to date. For other families, including those who have children who may become anxious just walking into the clinic or who have especially active children, a Drive-Up model for vaccine administration may be appealing. Within the community, gathering areas may serve as a point of familiarity, lowering the barrier to vaccination. Schools are logical partners, especially in efforts to reduce student school absences due to vaccine-preventable illness.[33]

Vaccine confidence starts with leadership, communication, and education
Achieving success with vaccination efforts starts with a commitment to the health of the patients, science, the scientific method, and to transparency. Leaders have the responsibility to set the stage of why vaccinating patients is of critical importance for the clinic, what outcomes will be measured, and sharing those outcomes regularly. The clinic culture of ensuring all staff, those directly involved in vaccination efforts and those indirectly involved, understand what their role is in promoting vaccination confidence is paramount. Education must be tailored to these distinct roles to allow each to fully be successful in their part of building a path to patient vaccination outcomes. Scorecards for physicians and nurse practitioners can take the abstract concept of patient vaccination rates to an actionable, patient-specific level.

The Role of the Pediatric Office Clinician and Staff in Building Vaccine Confidence

Vaccination's foundation is trust—strategies to build it
Vaccine hesitancy and misinformation must be fought not only with accurate and easily understandable information but also with trust. Trust is built on long-standing relationships grounded in humility, listening to one another, understanding what is important to each and why, authenticity, genuine caring, partnerships, and time. From within the clinic, vaccine champions in all roles, partnered with community advocates, can set the stage for a collaborative foundation.[34] Families who have stories of success, of overcoming fear, or who have experienced a vaccine preventable disease are voices that may be more trusted by hesitant families.[35]

Presumptive communication and other methods
There are several communication strategies staff in pediatric offices can use to raise vaccination rates as Limaye and colleagues[36] describe. Time is often the greatest barrier to effective communication, thus coordinating the proper appointment time is critical. These successful evidence-based communication strategies include the presumptive communication model to approach the conversation. Some experts recommend simply saying, "I am vaccinated, and I want you to be too," which Healy and Pickering[37] describe as the power of the "provider endorsement." With special scheduling for a longer conversation, the motivational interview[38] can be used, which is patient focused on a specific objective, for example, *I think my baby's immune system is too weak for vaccines and I need to understand that better before I vaccinate.*

Staff who are informed, open and able to discuss vaccines based on science and evidence on how to keep up

Pediatric offices are often limited in funds and time for continuing education for all staff. A well-educated staff promotes vaccine confidence among its patients. Following are suggestions for offices on how to stay abreast of ever-changing vaccine updates and the latest information:

- National conferences: some excellent conferences for all disciplines include the National Foundation for Infectious Diseases Clinical Vaccinology Course[15] and regular webinars at no cost, the CDC's National Immunization Conference,[16] and the Pediatric Infectious Disease annual conference in New York City.[17]
- Regional or local conferences: check with the state health department or state immunization coalition[18] for affordable conferences.
- On-line education: sign up for CDC email notification for webinars, information, summaries, and slide sets from their Clinician Outreach and Communication Activity (COCA) calls.[39] Use the interactive PIDS online Comprehensive Vaccine Education Program, at no charge even for nonmembers (https://pids.org/education-training/vaccine-education-program/).
- Publications: in addition to usual journals, pediatric practices should keep a current copy of *The Pinkbook, Epidemiology and Prevention of Vaccine-Preventable Diseases*[40] published by the CDC and found at https://www.cdc.gov/vaccines/pubs/pinkbook/index.html, which is a must for all practices.
- Reliable immunization Web site samples include the following:
  - CDC's COVID-1 Web site, www.vaccines.gov.[41]
  - Children's Hospital of Philadelphia's comprehensive Vaccine Education Center[42] is always timely at https://www.chop.edu/centers-programs/vaccine-education-center.
  - Immunize.org[18] has comprehensive, detailed immunization practice tips at http://www.immunize.org/. Especially helpful are the weekly emails one can request at www.immunize.org/express.
  - The National Foundation for Infectious Diseases[43] at http://www.nfid.org/ has in-depth Call-to-Action pieces on current immunization topics, infographics, and short public service announcements professionally made in English and Spanish that can be downloaded for use in the pediatric office.

Parents' Role in Achieving Vaccine Confidence

Parent responsibilities

Pediatric offices are unique in that there is not a single patient but a family with a pediatric patient who is developmentally changing at each visit and therefore needs a specialized approach. Although this can be challenging for the office staff, the responsibility to keep up with the immunization schedule is a shared one with whomever the patient defines as family. The caregiver must understand their state school-entry immunization laws and plan accordingly before school enrollment. Caregivers should prepare for the office visit by bringing all immunization records from clinics where the child may have been previously vaccinated. They have a responsibility to maintain immunization records on each child either by carrying a hard copy card or by enrolling in the office patient portal so records can be accessed electronically. Caregivers should allow clinics to enter their child's immunization data in the state's vaccine registry so if they move offices the data are available to the new pediatric provider; this prevents overvaccination, confusion, and frustration and delay at well-child visits. It is the caregiver's responsibility to read the federally required vaccine information statement[44] from the CDC before each vaccination. If a parent is unable to read or does not understand content, they need to speak up and ask staff questions on behalf of their child, and staff must be open and prepared for this at each encounter. Parents must never threaten their children with vaccinations as a punishment in a clinic setting, but instead should praise their child for participating in one of the best health promoting functions of all. Parents and guardians can play a vital role in how the vaccination experience goes by preparing the child or teen before the visit in an age-appropriate manner. Kids of all ages benefit from distraction either by watching a kids' video or by listening to music with headphones to pass the prevaccination time, which can be stressful. Praise, rewards, and a special treat together with the newly vaccinated child is an important parent role in making the vaccination experience a positive one.

Understanding where and how to find reliable resources

Getting good, evidence-based, reliable vaccine resources is more challenging than ever for parents of children due to the amount of misinformation and disinformation on social media that is difficult to distinguish from credible educational material. Parents can use the Web sites noted earlier, most of which have sections accessible to parents. Vaccinate Your Family,[45] an immunization advocacy group, developed a helpful guide called *Immunization Resources for Parents and Parents-To-Be* in collaboration with the US Department of Agriculture[46] in English and Spanish and can be found at https://wicworks.fns.usda.gov/resources/immunization-resources-parents-and-parents-be. In addition, professional associations that specialize in the care of children and adolescents offer reliable social media sites, such as the National Association of Pediatric Nurse Practitioners (NAPNAP)[47] at https://kidshealth.org/NAPNAP/en/parents and the American Academy of Pediatricians (AAP)[48] at https://healthychildren.org/, whose resources include Spanish language information.

Public relations campaigns to drive support in clinic conversations

From a family culture to a pediatric office culture to our larger societal community, we must all do our part to reduce vaccine preventable diseases. As part of a larger society, we have a social contract to agree to stop at red traffic lights, to not smoke cigarettes indoors or throw them onto dry lands, and to not drink and drive so that we make decisions to protect ourselves and others. Vaccination should be seen similarly: *when I protect my child, I protect your child.* Public relations campaigns have gotten us to understand these societal norms and can be used as a backdrop to pediatric office conversations about vaccination to drive support in the clinic conversation as a social norm. Pediatric office staff should help participate in developing appropriate messages, collaborating with their local and state health departments as they know their population best.

SUMMARY

Whether for annual influenza vaccine or primary series vaccines the following advice pertains:

"Vaccination rates may also be increased by interventions that increase patient demand and access to vaccines and overcome practice-related barriers. Such interventions include vaccination-only clinics, standing orders, strong recommendations from healthcare providers, as well as reminder and recall efforts. For maximum impact on immunization rates, interventions should be combined into a multifaceted immunization program rather than used alone. Interventions that address site-specific needs, taking resources into account, should be implemented on a practice-by-practice basis."[49]

Together, the complex operational endeavor of pediatric vaccination, one of the most life-saving endeavors of all, can be realized with vaccine confidence, successful, safe vaccination resulting in reduction of vaccine preventable diseases.

CLINICAL PEARLS

- Patient safety and continuous quality improvement principles can be used to optimize immunization rates in pediatric practices.
- An engaged team with clear roles within an office culture of safety and strong leadership who values vaccination will improve their clinic's vaccination rates.
- Missed opportunities to vaccinate can be reduced with multipronged strategies such as reminder-recall processes, using standing orders, having daily vaccine huddles, and considering every visit a vaccine visit.
- A dedicated "Vaccine Specialist" is a critical role to optimizing vaccination best practices in the pediatric office setting.
- Recognition that pain results in fear and stress can depress vaccine compliance rates; thus, minimizing pain through proven methods increases adherence and family satisfaction scores.
- Institutional and unrecognized bias are pervasive in society and medicine; vaccine programs are no different and require diverse voices to be engaged to address equity issues that may not be recognized; start by hiring staff from the cultures served.
- When hesitant families ultimately choose to vaccinate, the staff are ready with properly stored, handled, and administered vaccines providing comfort techniques that promote vaccine confidence for future return vaccinations.

DISCLOSURE

No authors have any relevant conflicts of interest to disclose.

REFERENCES

1. Stokley S, Kempe A, Stockwell MS, et al. Improving pediatric vaccination coverage in the United States. Acad Pediatr 2021;21(4):S1–2.
2. Freed GL, Clark SJ, Butchart AT, et al. Sources and perceived credibility of vaccine-safety information for parents. Pediatrics 2011;127(Suppl 1):S107–12.
3. Offit PA, DeStefano F. Vaccine safety. Vaccines 2013;1464–80. https://doi.org/10.1016/B978-1-4557-0090-5.00076-8.
4. Reason J. Human error: models and management. Br Med J 2009;320:768–70.
5. Shah V, Taddio A, Rieder MJ, HELPinKIDS Team. Effectiveness and tolerability of pharmacologic and combined interventions for reducing injection pain during routine childhood immunizations: systematic review and meta-analyses. Clin Ther 2009;31(Suppl 2):S104–51.
6. Friedrichsdorf SJ, Eull D, Weidner C, et al. A hospital-wide initiative to eliminate or reduce needle pain in children using lean methodology. Pain Rep 2018;3(Suppl 1):e671.
7. The Children's Comfort Promise video (YouTube link The Children's Minnesota Comfort Promise).https://m.youtube.com/watch?v=-awNlwMQ6nA.
8. Doyle R, Donaldson A, Philips L, et al. The impact of a multidisciplinary care package for vaccination in needle phobic children: an observational study. J Paediatr Child Health 2022;58(7):1174–80.

9. US Centers for Disease Control and Prevention. Vaccine Adverse Event Reporting System (VAERS). Available at: https://vaers.hhs.gov/. Accessed May 29, 2022.
10. Borchardt SM, Mitchell K, Larson T, et al. Applying the AFIX quality improvement model to increase adult immunization in Wisconsin. Public Health Rep 2021; 136(5):603–8.
11. Paoli S, Lorini C, Puggelli F, et al. Assessing vaccine hesitancy among healthcare workers: a cross-sectional study at an Italian paediatric hospital and the development of a healthcare worker's vaccination compliance index. Vaccine 2019; 7(4):201.
12. Li A.J., Tabu C., Shendale S., et al., Qualitative insights into reasons for missed opportunities for vaccination in Kenyan health facilities, PLoS One, 15 (3), 2020, e0230783.
13. Centers for Disease Control and Prevention (CDC). Vaccine storage and handling resources. 2021. Available at: https://www.cdc.gov/vaccines/hcp/admin/storage/index.html. Accessed June 2, 2022.
14. You must provide patients with vaccine information statements (VISs) – It's Federal Law!. 2022. Available at: https://www.immunize.org/catg.d/p2027.pdf. Accessed June 2, 2022.
15. National Foundation for Infectious Diseases Clinical Vaccinology Course. Available at: https://cvc.nfid.org/. Accessed June 14, 2022.
16. Centers for Disease Control and Prevention. National Immunization Conference. Available at: https://www.cdc.gov/vaccines/events/nic/index.html. Accessed June 14, 2022.
17. Infectious Diseases in Children Symposium. New York City. Available at: https://www.healio.com/meeting/idcnewyork/home. Accessed June 14, 2022.
18. Immunize.org, formerly Immunization Action Coalition. Available at: www.immunize.org. State Coalitions. Accessed June 14, 2022.
19. Sampath B, Rakover J, Baldoza K, et al. Whole system quality: a unified approach to building responsive, resilient health care systems. IHI White Paper. Boston: Institute for Healthcare Improvement; 2021.
20. Rand CM, Humiston SG. Provider focused interventions to improve child and adolescent vaccination rates. Acad Pediatr 2021;21(4):S34–9.
21. Jaca A., Mathebula L., Iweze, A., et al., A systematic review of strategies for reducing missed opportunities for vaccination, Vaccine, 36 (21), 2018, 2921–2927.
22. Stockwell MS, Stokley S, Kempe A. Implementing effective vaccination interventions into sustainable 'real world' practice. Acad Pediatr 2021;21(4): S78–80.
23. Proctor EK, Powell BJ, McMillen JC. Implementation strategies: recommendations for specifying and reporting. Implement Sci 2013;8:139.
24. Langley GJ, Nolan KM, Nolan TW, et al. The improvement guide: a practical approach to enhancing organizational performance. 2nd edition. San Francisco (CA): Jossey-Bass; 2009. p. 24.
25. Hargreaves A.L., Nowak G., Frew, P., et al., Adherence to timely vaccinations in the United States, Pediatrics, 145 (3), 2020, e20190783.
26. Mueller BU, Adirim T, Franklin W, et al, Council on Quality Improvement and Patient Safety, Committee on Hospital Care. Principles ofs. Pediatrics 2019;143(2): e20183649.
27. Wolicki J. and Miller E., Vaccine administration, In: Hall E., Wodi A.P., Hamborsky J., et al., Epidemiology and prevention of vaccine-preventable diseases. 14th edition.

Centers for Disease Control and Prevention, 2021, Public Health Foundation; Washington, DC. Available at: https://www.cdc.gov/vaccines/pubs/pinkbook/vac-admin.html, Accessed June 2, 2022. 72-73.

28. National Foundation for Infectious Disease. Clinical Vaccinology Course. Available at: https://cvc.nfid.org/. Accessed June 2, 2022.
29. National Center for Immunization and Respiratory Diseases. Vaccine storage and handling toolkit. 2022. Available at: https://www.cdc.gov/vaccines/hcp/admin/storage/toolkit/index.html. Accessed June 2, 2022.
30. Greenfield LS, Page L, et al. Strategies for increasing adolescent immunizations in diverse ethnic communities. J Adolesc Health 2015;56(5 Suppl):S47–53.
31. Ma A, Sanchez A, Ma M, et al. The impact of patient-provider race/ethnicity concordance on provider visits: updated evidence from the medical expenditure panel survey. J Racial Ethn Health Disparities 2019;6:1011–20.
32. Gellin B, Maibach E, et al. Do Parents Understand Immunizations? A National Telephone Survey. Pediatrics 2000;106(5):1097–102.
33. Cawley J., Hull H.F., Rousculp, M.D., Strategies for Implementing school-located influenza vaccination of children: a systematic literature review, J Sch Health, 80, 2010, 167–175.
34. Willis E, Sabnis S, et al. Improving immunization rates through community-based participatory research: community health improvement for Milwaukee's Children Program. Prog Community Health Partnersh 2010;10(1):19–30.
35. Cunningham R.M. and Boom J.A., Telling stories of vaccine-preventable diseases: why it works. *S D Med.* 2013;Spec no:21-26.
36. Limaye RJ, Opel DJ, Dempsey A, et al. Communicating with vaccine-hesitant parents: a narrative review. Acad Pediatr 2021;21(4):S24–9.
37. Healy CM, Pickering LK. How to communicate with vaccine-hesitant parents. Pediatrics 2011;127(Suppl 1):S127–33.
38. World Health Organization. Motivational interviewing. Available at: www.WHO.int/immunization/programmes_systems/Training Module_ConversationGuide_final.pptx. Accessed May 29, 2022.
39. Centers for Disease Control and Prevention. Clinician Outreach and Communication Activities, (COCA) Calls. Available at: https://emergency.cdc.gov/coca/. Accessed June 14, 2022.
40. Epidemiology and Prevention of Vaccine-Preventable Diseases, The Pink Book: Course Textbook - 14th edition. 2021. Available at: https://www.cdc.gov/vaccines/pubs/pinkbook/index.html.
41. Centers for Disease Control and Prevention Vaccines. Available at: www.vaccines.gov. Accessed May 26, 2022.
42. Children's Hospital of Philadelphia, Vaccine Education Center. Available at: https://www.chop.edu/centers-programs/vaccine-education-center. Accessed May 26, 2022.
43. National Foundation for Infectious Diseases. Available at: www.nfid.org. Accessed June 14, 2022.
44. Centers for Disease Control and Prevention. Vaccine Information Statements. Available at: https://www.cdc.gov/vaccines/hcp/vis/index.html. Accessed June 14, 2022.
45. Vaccinate Your Family. Available at: https://vaccinateyourfamily.org/. Accessed June 14, 2022.
46. Immunization Resources for Parents and Parents-To-Be. Vaccinate Your Family and US Department of Agriculture. Available at: https://wicworks.fns.usda.gov/

resources/immunization-resources-parents-and-parents-be. Accessed May 26, 2022.

47. National Association of Pediatric Nurse Practitioners (NAPNAP). Available at: https://kidshealth.org/NAPNAP/en/parents. Accessed May 26, 2022.

48. American Academy of Pediatrics (AAP). Available at: www.shopaap.org. Accessed May 26, 2022.

49. Stinchfield PK. Practice-proven interventions to increase vaccination rates and broaden the immunization season. Am J Med 2008;121(7 Suppl 2):S11–21.

Overcoming Vaccine Hesitancy Using Community-Based Efforts

Lori E. Crosby, PsyD[a,b,*], Francis J. Real, MD, MEd[b,c],
Jodi Cunnigham, PhD[d], Monica Mitchell, PhD[a,b,e]

KEYWORDS

- Pediatrics • Vaccine hesitancy • Vaccination • Immunization • Community settings
- Vaccine communication • Community engagement

KEY POINTS

- Community-based strategies can augment clinical vaccine hesitancy interventions.
- Community-level assessment of vaccine hesitancy and barriers that engages and is led by trusted community key stakeholders is critical to developing effective interventions.
- Tailored communication strategies including training parents/caregivers and community leaders as vaccine champions holds promise.
- Partnering with health departments, schools, and pharmacies is an effective strategy for overcoming parent/caregiver vaccine hesitancy and improving access to childhood vaccinations.

BACKGROUND

Each year millions of children and adolescents experience vaccine-preventable diseases due to low vaccine acceptance by parents and other caregivers. Many factors contribute to vaccine hesitancy or "the motivational state of being conflicted about or opposed to getting vaccinated"[1] including misinformation about vaccines and social and structural barriers (In Francis J. Real and colleagues' article, "Using Technology to Overcome Vaccine Hesitancy," in this issue) to vaccine access.[2] Vaccine hesitancy

[a] Division of Behavioral Medicine, Cincinnati Children's Hospital Medical Center, 3333 Burnet Avenue, MLC 7039, Cincinnati, OH 45229, USA; [b] Department of Pediatrics, University of Cincinnati College of Medicine, Cincinnati, OH, USA; [c] Division of General and Community Pediatrics, Cincinnati Children's Hospital Medical Center, 3333 Burnet Avenue, MLC 2011, Cincinnati, OH 45229, USA; [d] The Community Builders, Inc., 3635 Reading Road, Cincinnati, OH 45229, USA; [e] Community Relations, Cincinnati Children's Hospital Medical Center, 3333 Burnet Avenue, MLC 7039, Cincinnati, OH 45229, USA
* Corresponding author. Division of Behavioral Medicine, Cincinnati Children's Hospital Medical Center, 3333 Burnet Avenue, MLC 7039, Cincinnati, OH 45229.
E-mail address: Lori.Crosby@cchmc.org

Pediatr Clin N Am 70 (2023) 359–370
https://doi.org/10.1016/j.pcl.2022.11.012
0031-3955/23/© 2022 Elsevier Inc. All rights reserved.
pediatric.theclinics.com

sits on a continuum from refusal to acceptance with unique influences for each caregiver or individual. One caregiver may have concerns about side effects, whereas another may be more concerned that the vaccine was rushed or may not be effective. This article reviews key challenges and advantages of evidence-based community strategies for overcoming parent/caregiver vaccine hesitancy including community-participatory vaccine hesitancy measurement, communication approaches, reinforcement techniques (eg, incentives, mandates), and community-engaged partnerships.

Community-level assessment of barriers to combatting vaccine hesitancy is an essential first step to increase vaccination rates, although data in isolation are insufficient to support effective intervention development. Involving families and key stakeholders in the review of community data and identification of concerns is vital to inform messaging and intervention planning. Caregivers and stakeholders possess unique insights into what might work for whom (ie, who needs to hear what), how messages can be delivered most effectively (ie, from whom and where), and the best ways to manage misinformation (ie, what to ignore and what to address).

Within communities, misinformation about vaccines can increase hesitancy.[1] Many caregivers rely on social media or online searches for health information. Indeed, approximately 84% of Americans view vaccine-related Web pages annually.[3] However, search engines frequently return Web pages critical of vaccination that are of lower quality than noncritical Web pages.[4] Moreover, most individuals are unaware that dotcom sites have a commercial designation and, therefore, may not always feature evidence-based information especially if it conflicts with their product, service, or profit margin. Social media has been found to play a key role in spreading health misinformation by providing a largely unregulated backdrop for antivaccine messages to propagate, which is notable because nearly half of US adults report obtaining vaccine information through social media.[5] Tailored communication strategies such as virtual town hall series offer opportunities to assess current myths or misinformation that caregivers may be exposed to in real time before myths gain traction within communities. Furthermore, engagement in community discussions or conversations with trusted community leaders offer caregivers the opportunity to hear other caregivers' concerns and have their individual concerns addressed.

Many communities have instituted vaccine mandates related to school attendance for children and adolescents. Data support that mandates can be an effective strategy for increasing coverage for childhood and adolescent vaccinations; however, the use of reinforcement techniques (positive or negative) is tricky because it can negatively influence parent/caregiver autonomy and future vaccination decisions. Most childhood vaccines are given at pediatric primary care offices, yet we know that not all children have access to a high-quality primary care medical home.[6,7] Those with access may also face challenges related to accessing care such as limited operating clinic hours during evenings and weekends as well as transportation problems.[2] Moreover, due to competing work or personal demands, some families prioritize acute care over primary care. Offering vaccinations in collaboration with partners in community settings (eg, schools, pharmacies) is a promising strategy that may address barriers to accessing vaccines for some families.[2]

Community-Participatory Measurement

Identifying and measuring barriers to vaccine hesitancy is a critical first step in developing effective community-based vaccine hesitancy interventions. Such data may be obtained through meaningful interactions with community members and obtained during health events, health fairs, and school meetings among other venues. Existing tools focus on measuring parent hesitancy toward childhood and adolescent vaccination (Parent Attitudes about Childhood Vaccines survey[8] and the Vaccine Confidence Scale[9,10]) or psychological antecedents (eg, collective responsibility) that impact vaccine decisions (5C Scale[11]). However, in response to the coronavirus disease 2019 (COVID-19) pandemic, several new tools measuring parental vaccine attitudes, intentions, and behaviors are being developed and evaluated. For example, the Vaccine Barriers Assessment Tool[12] that assesses barriers to childhood vaccination including access to vaccination is being evaluated in New Zealand and Australia. If found to be beneficial at assessing acceptance and external barriers, it could be adapted for use in the United States. Furthermore, the World Health Organization (WHO) Working Group on the Behavioral and Social Drivers of vaccination is developing tools to measure the drivers of vaccination. In addition, the Kaiser Family Foundation (KFF) regularly assesses parental attitudes and intentions about COVID-19 vaccination including ranking the top reported influential factors along with national COVID-19 childhood vaccination rates. Of note, a report from the KFF from April 2022 that assessed the perspectives of 1889 adults (including 501 Hispanic individuals and 500 non-Hispanic black individuals) identified an adult's doctor or child's pediatrician as the most trusted resource for information about the COVID-19 vaccine.[13] KFF displays current data on their Web site with an option to download it. It is notable that parents who do not intend to vaccinate their children have participated in KFF surveys, supporting the use of these types of tools for assessing the perspectives of a range of parents along the vaccine hesitancy continuum. KFF's recommended community-engaged practice of presenting data back to the community fosters transparency and builds trust.[14] Thus, this practice may result in parents feeling validated and open to changing their stance as they see the number of parents reporting concerns and barriers over time decrease mirroring changes in vaccination rates.

Hood and colleagues[15] are using a mobile app to collect real-time data on parental attitudes about COVID-19 vaccination, including attitudes about having their children vaccinated. This study is being conducted in the United Kingdom, United States, and Mexico and involves community advisory boards who give input on both the questions asked and what and how data are displayed. Similarly, but specific to adolescents, Rosen and colleagues[16] used intervention mapping, a systematic process to engage stakeholders in intervention development, to create a virtual reality (VR) curriculum to support clinicians' communication skills when recommending the COVID-19 vaccine.[17] Parent involvement in the assessment of vaccine hesitancy and barriers ensures that the right questions are asked to help identify the reasons parents may delay or decline vaccination. Data from these measures can be used to develop communication strategies and are integral to designing tailored intervention strategies to improve uptake of child and adolescent vaccines.

Communication Approaches

To reach marginalized or communities of color, community-based approaches to vaccination involve both broad public health campaigns to promote childhood vaccination and tailored messaging, or health messaging designed consistent with individual or group characteristics.[1,18] Tailored messaging involves (1) use of communication methods most frequently used by a group or subpopulation (eg, the social medial platform used may differ by age group, racial/ethnic identity), (2) having images representative of the population (eg, diverse images particularly if there is stigma associated with the vaccination as in the case of sexually transmitted diseases), (3) use of appropriate language, and (4) honoring diversity within subpopulations and ensuring messages are meaningful.[18] When developed with input from parents or communities, communication tools (eg, flyers, social media posts, blogs,

Web site posts, videos) can directly address common myths (ie, debunk misinformation) and provide alternative explanations that can be used in future discussions about childhood vaccination with family members or friends. Active promotion of influenza vaccination via visual displays or media campaigns has been reported as a motivating factor for some individuals to seek out vaccination.[19] The degree of impact of media campaigns might be related to its perceived credibility by the target community.[20] Likewise, messages delivered by media outlets have the potential to negatively impact vaccine perceptions in communities. For example, political and gendered messaging have likely negatively impacted the public's understanding of the human papillomavirus (HPV) vaccine.[21] Similarly, COVID-19 vaccine intention has been influenced by partisan media use.[22] As such, the COVID-19 pandemic has underscored the importance of developing evidence-based methods and systems to supportive vaccine confidence relevant to specific communities.[22] For example, Jensen and colleagues[23] developed short video-based messages to nudge COVID-19 vaccine intentions and showed a decrease in vaccine hesitancy. Similarly, Crosby and Rule[24] developed tailored videos for the black and Latino populations in Cincinnati, OH, and their qualitative results indicated that participants who viewed the videos reported increased vaccine confidence. Posting tailored communication tools in venues where parents live, work, play, and visit (eg, Web sites, social media platforms) increases the likelihood that parents will be exposed to accurate information and messages that support childhood vaccination. Ultimately, such clear and accessible information empowers parents and caregivers to make advantageous choices to support their child(ren)'s health.[25]

Tailored messaging approaches may be even more effective when paired with community discussions or town halls. One of the major advantages of these town hall discussions is that parents can get their specific concerns addressed real time. In addition, they can hear aloud what other parents are considering as they make decisions about vaccination.

To be most effective, town hall speakers should include trusted members of the community and be prepared to respond to vaccine critics. The WHO has recommended a 3-step process for addressing criticism in a public forum.[26]

1. Step 1 is to name the tactic (eg, cherry picking evidence)
2. Step 2 is to identify the topic (eg, low threat of disease)
3. Step 3 is to respond with a key message that unmasks the technique related to the topic (eg, "There is overwhelming scientific evidence showing that vaccination saves millions of lives every year. Vaccination is one of the most successful and cost-effective public health interventions.").[26]

During the COVID-19 pandemic, many town halls switched to a virtual format increasing their frequency and expanding their reach. However, town halls may be most beneficial for parents who have already made the decision to vaccinate or are strongly considering vaccination. Additional strategies are needed to reach parents with serious vaccination concerns or negative attitudes toward vaccination. Moreover, most of these programs are designed for primarily US-born English-speaking families and may not meet the needs of parents who are from different cultures or experience language barriers. Innovative technology may support reach to vulnerable families. For example, Streuli and colleagues[27] used community-based participatory research methods to develop a culturally and linguistically appropriate VR (see Douglas J. Opel's article, "Clinician Communication to Address Vaccine Hesitancy," in this issue) vaccination program for a refugee community, which is being evaluated to determine its impact on vaccine attitudes and intentions.

The use of vaccine champions or trusted messengers, alongside communication campaigns, is a valuable community-based strategy for overcoming hesitancy.[1] The Centers for Disease Control and Prevention have specifically identified use of vaccine recipients and trusted messengers as a critical component of their framework to support vaccination in the United States, entitled *Vaccinate with Confidence.*[28] Vaccine champions may be community leaders, caretakers, pharmacy students, or health care providers who are trained to understand childhood vaccination (what they are, how vaccines are developed, vaccine schedules, side effects, and so on) and equipped with accurate information to address specific vaccination concerns. Interventions aiming to increase vaccine uptake have traditionally focused on medical providers given the well-described impact of their strong recommendations on vaccination rates (see Ashley B Stephens and colleagues' article, "Influenza Vaccine Hesitancy: Scope, Influencing Factors, and Strategic Interventions"; and E. Adrianne Hammershaimb and colleagues' article, "COVID-19 Vaccine Hesitancy"; and Jennifer D. Kusma and colleagues' article, "A Structural Lens Approach to Vaccine Hesitancy and Identity"; and Amisha Malhotra and Patricia Whitley-Williams' article, "Training Residents and Medical Students to Overcome Parents' Vaccine Hesitancy," in this issue).[10,29] VR simulation has been used to effectively train health care providers in messaging practices and might have applicability for training community champions.[30] For example, Cincinnati Children's Hospital is using group-based VR to train nurses, staff, and pharmacists to address vaccine hesitancy prior in preparation for working with families at a community-based influenza vaccine event. Combining strong recommendations with personal stories from vaccine champions can be a powerful tool for combating vaccine hesitancy by supporting consistent, positive messaging. In person and on social media, such champions can share consistent, positive messages related to vaccination within their communities to support uptake.

Vaccine champions may positively impact social norms and build parental confidence in vaccination. Vaccination is an "invisible" behavior so caregivers may not know how common it is; also, because vaccine hesitancy gets more attention, caregivers may assume that it is more common.[31] Vaccine champions can inform caregivers about the high rates of vaccination, thereby, increasing the "visibility" or normality of this behavior. One example of a vaccine champion approach using community leaders is described by Sims and colleagues[32]; they report increased influenza vaccination rates at a community health event where faith-based leaders communicated the importance of getting vaccinated and then received the vaccine in front of attendees. Another example in which parents/caregivers served as vaccine champions is the "Immunity Community" campaign; parents/caregivers were trained to become immunization advocates and engage other parents/caregivers in discussions about vaccination.[33] Data revealed a decrease in the proportion of vaccine-hesitant participants. Similarly, Colorado Parents for Vaccinated Communities is a community-based project initiated by the Colorado Children's Immunization Coalition that also engages parents in advocacy around vaccination.[34] This approach has also been used for the COVID-19 vaccine (see Cynthia M. Rand and Courtney Olson-Chen's article, "Maternal Vaccination and Vaccine Hesitancy," in this issue). For instance, a COVID-19 Vaccine Champions and Communication program initially developed in Australia is being adapted for use in Western countries.[35] Community-based efforts like these that harness the voices of parents and community leaders to address vaccine hesitancy help to reinforce vaccination as a social norm.

Reinforcement Techniques

Some communities, health insurance, and managed care companies use incentives to reinforce childhood vaccinations. Within this approach, parents may receive cash prizes, gift cards, drawings, or discounts as rewards for having their child vaccinated. A free weekly lottery (Vax-a-Million) for individuals who received at least 1 COVID-19 vaccine in Ohio resulted in 114,554 additional Ohioans being vaccinated when compared with a control site at the cost of $49 per additional vaccinated individual.[36] A study in Sweden also demonstrated a positive impact of monetary incentives on COVID-19 vaccination rates.[37] However, a systematic review in 2013 found insufficient evidence to support incentives, particularly financial incentives. Incentive rewards such as government payments, lottery prizes, gift cards, and food vouchers must be carefully considered to avoid coercion of vulnerable populations. These types of programs may have unintended consequences; they could support stigmatization of those individuals who choose not to participate and could reduce uptake in the future when the incentives disappear.[38] Additional studies are needed to understand how incentives might best support vaccine uptake.[39,40]

Other institutions (schools, workplaces) have used mandates in which individuals are penalized or denied services for not vaccinating. For example, many schools require childhood and some adolescent immunizations be completed before school enrollment. It is notable that some mandates receive very little pushback (eg, mandate to have a license to drive), whereas others such as child/adolescent immunizations or the COVID-19 vaccine may be challenged. Although most vaccine mandates are state driven, mandates by independent federal agencies such as the Occupational Safety and Health Administration tend to have a broader impact.[41] Data suggest that mandates do increase vaccination coverage particularly when the baseline rate is low.[42] However, causality is complex.[43] Communities often use multiple strategies to improve vaccination rates, so it is difficult to know if an increase is related to the combination or a single strategy. Mandates may have significant unintended consequences from stigma to worsening inequities and eroding trust.[44] Mandates may also make parents more committed to their decision to not vaccinate if the perception is that vaccination will decrease personal control over their health care decisions for their children.[40]

Community-Engaged Partnerships

Research suggests that partnering with community-based (eg, community-based health) organizations, health (eg, public health departments), education (eg, historically black college and universities), civic corporations (eg, sororities, fraternities), faith-based organizations (eg, churches, collaboratives), and social agencies (eg, county health and mental health agencies) to overcome parental vaccination hesitancy is a best practice.[2] The literature provides numerous examples of partnerships between public health departments and primary care physicians, public health departments and schools, community pharmacies and community organizations, and so on to offer educational events and vaccines in community settings. These partnerships are effective because community partners may be trusted sources for parents, can reach large numbers of parents and families, and have resources (staff, incentives) that make vaccination convenient and feasible for parents and families. Overall, these strategies have resulted in increased vaccination coverage.[45] The National Vaccine Advisory Committee recommends partnerships, such as between health departments and schools, to improve delivery of immunizations and overcome barriers (goals 4 and 5). The committee has also developed quality standards for vaccine administration outside of primary care offices (eg, schools, pharmacies, community events).[46]

One key advantage to offering vaccination in community settings is the convenience and the ability to meet children and families where they are. For parents, this could mean getting their own vaccine and having all of their children vaccinated simultaneously. Home visits have been found to be effective for increasing childhood vaccination rates when used in combination with other interventions such as parent education, telephone/automated reminders, and case management.[47–49] Such offering of vaccination to all household members has been an effective approach to supporting COVID-19 vaccination even within clinical settings.[50] Another advantage to vaccination in community settings is that these sites bring vaccination to where viruses/diseases live, in the community; this is important given the need to reach populations who may have challenges related to accessibility, transportation, and trust. Thus, motivation to vaccinate might be prompted by community-based messaging from trusted entities.

Schools/childcare centers are an important community setting where vaccination might occur.[45] Vaccines are administered in schools using 1 of 2 models: (1) school-based health centers or (2) temporary vaccine clinics in schools.[2,51] School-based health centers often serve as medical homes for youth who experience geographic, financial, or cultural barriers to accessing care.[52] Typically, in urban or rural settings, they provide preventative medical care to youth who are often considered hard to reach.[53] A large randomized controlled trial in the city of Rochester, New York, demonstrated a small though statistically significant increase in influenza vaccination rates among adolescents with availability of school-located influenza vaccination programs.[54] However, not all schools have school-based health centers and existing school-based health centers do not always have the resources to provide immunizations.[55] In addition, not all students enrolled in a specific school will receive care at their school-based health center.[52]

Most temporary school vaccine clinics focus on the influenza vaccine, and these efforts have resulted in increased uptake.[54] In collaboration with public health partners, school clinics have also been very effective at immunizing children during outbreaks.[52] Owing to the temporary nature of these clinics, there are challenges with obtaining parental consent, verifying insurance, and coordination with the primary care office to notify them that the child was vaccinated at school. In addition, these clinics require buy-in from the school district because they can be costly.[44]

Pharmacies are another important community setting for vaccination; in fact, they can be part of a child's "immunization neighborhood."[56] Indeed, adolescent influenza immunization administration rates within pharmacies have increased leading to recommendations for them to provide HPV vaccination within their setting.[2] Pharmacists have played and will continue to play a key role in administration of the COVID-19 vaccine for both adults and children.[57] Caregiver familiarity with local pharmacies and the convenience of having their child vaccinated simultaneously make this a preferred option for some caregivers. Although pharmacy administration of childhood vaccines is an important strategy to increase uptake, parents must also consider their comfort level with the limited confidentiality at a community pharmacy.

Although effective, offering vaccines in community settings creates some challenges. For example, maintaining an adequate supply of vaccine can be difficult when the number of children who need vaccines is unknown.[2] Storing the temperature-sensitive vaccine can also be a limiting factor. Venues may not be set up with storage space or freezers to store vaccines. Partnerships with health departments are beneficial because insurance reimbursement for vaccines in community settings is often insufficient. Staffing can also be a challenge because events may rely on volunteers who could feel uncomfortable with having vaccination conversations without specific training. Staff may also have difficulty accessing child vaccination records particularly if they are not entered into an electronic statewide system.

SUMMARY

The drivers of vaccine hesitancy are varied; thus, a critical first step to developing community-based interventions is to identify the unique barriers for parents, caregivers, and communities. Tailoring vaccine communication campaigns to be context specific increases their relevance and ability to guide parents toward change. In addition, parent confidence in immunizations may increase through discussions with "vaccine champions" or trusted messengers who are from the community. Although incentives and mandates have been shown to increase vaccination coverage, these strategies may have unintended consequences for parents and caretakers (ie, undermine trust, reinforce vaccine hesitancy). Engaging trusted partners (eg, town halls, faith-based communities, civic organizations) to address misinformation and improving access (eg, schools, health departments, pharmacies, mobile clinics) may be the most effective community-based approaches to overcome parental vaccine hesitancy.

CLINICS CARE POINTS

- Pediatric health and primary care practices and providers play a critical role in ensuring that children are vaccinated. It is important that primary care providers partner with community allies (health departments, schools, faith-based organizations, civic organizations, pharmacies, and so on) to overcome barriers related to vaccine access and vaccine hesitancy.

- Pediatric health and primary care providers can incorporate messages in clinical materials that help parents and caregivers understand information about vaccines and options for their children. Some of these messages should be developed by community groups. This will build trust and reduce the potential for misunderstanding and misinformation. Providing links to reliable, timely, and accurate sources of information with attention to reaching diverse audiences is important. Translated materials are needed to reflect the communities served.

- It is recommended that pediatric health and primary care providers participate in continuing education as needed to be knowledgeable on vaccinations, and in ways to answer parents' questions about emerging issues related to pediatric and adolescent vaccinations and guidelines. Community and cultural sensitivity are also important when building trust and addressing vaccine hesitancy.

- Pediatric health and primary care providers can serve on panels with parents, caregivers, patients, and community members to provide expertise and gain feedback from valued community leaders and members on how to improve messaging, form collaborations, build trust and ultimately address vaccine hesitancy, increase vaccinations, and improve pediatric and adolescent health.

DISCLOSURE

The authors have nothing to disclose.

FUNDING

This work was supported in part by the CCTST at the University of Cincinnati which is funded by the National Institutes of Health (NIH) Clinical and Translational Science Award (CTSA) program, grant UL1TR001425.

REFERENCES

1. Tuckerman J, Kaufman J, Danchin M. Effective approaches to combat vaccine hesitancy. Pediatr Infect Dis J 2022;41(5):e243–5.

2. Hofstetter AM, Schaffer S. Childhood and adolescent vaccination in alternative settings. Acad Pediatr 2021;21(4):S50–6.
3. Guess AM, Nyhan B, O'Keeffe Z, et al. The sources and correlates of exposure to vaccine-related (mis)information online. Vaccine 2020;38(49):7799–805.
4. Fu LY, Zook K, Spoehr-Labutta Z, et al. Search engine ranking, quality, and content of web pages that are critical versus noncritical of human papillomavirus vaccine. J Adolesc Health 2016;58(1):33–9.
5. Mitchell A, Liedke J. About four-in-ten Americans say social media is an important way of following COVID-19 vaccine news. In Policy Commons. 2021. Available at: https://policycommons.net/artifacts/1808909/about-four-in-ten-americans-say-social-media-is-an-important-way-of-following-covid-19-vaccine-news/2543882/. Accessed June 1, 2022.
6. Wood DL. Increasing immunization coverage. American Academy of Pediatrics Committee on Community Health Services. American Academy of Pediatrics Committee on Practice and Ambulatory Medicine. Pediatrics 2003;112(4):993–6.
7. Rand CM, Goldstein NPN. Patterns of primary care physician visits for us adolescents in 2014: implications for vaccination. Acad Pediatr 2018;18(2, Supplement):S72–8.
8. Opel DJ, Taylor JA, Zhou C, et al. The relationship between parent attitudes about childhood vaccines survey scores and future child immunization status: a validation study. JAMA Pediatr 2013;167(11):1065–71.
9. Gilkey MB, Magnus BE, Reiter PL, et al. The Vaccination Confidence Scale: a brief measure of parents' vaccination beliefs. Vaccine 2014;32(47):6259–65.
10. Gilkey MB, Reiter PL, Magnus BE, et al. Validation of the vaccination confidence scale: a brief measure to identify parents at risk for refusing adolescent vaccines. Acad Pediatr 2016;16(1):42–9.
11. Betsch C, Schmid P, Heinemeier D, et al. Beyond confidence: Development of a measure assessing the 5C psychological antecedents of vaccination. PlOS ONE 2018;13(12):e0208601.
12. Kaufman J, Tuckerman J, Bonner C, et al. Parent-level barriers to uptake of childhood vaccination: a global overview of systematic reviews. BMJ Glob Health 2021;6(9):e006860.
13. Kaiser Family Foundation. KFF COVID-19 vaccine monitor April 2022. 2022. Available at: https://files.kff.org/attachment/TOPLINE-KFF-COVID-19-Vaccine-Monitor-April-2022.pdf. Accessed June 1, 2022.
14. Bodison SC, Sankaré I, Anaya H, et al. Engaging the community in the dissemination, implementation, and improvement of health-related research. Clin Translational Sci 2015;8(6):814–9.
15. Hood AM, Stotesbury H, Murphy J, et al. Attitudes about covid-19 and health (attach): Online survey and mixed methods study. JMIR Ment Health 2021; 8(10):e29963.
16. Rosen BL, Meisman A, Sun Q, et al. Factors Associated with Adolescents and Young Adults' Intention to Receive a COVID-19 Vaccine. J Adolesent Health 2022;70(4):S17.
17. Fernandez ME, Ruiter RA, Markham CM, et al. Intervention mapping: theory-and evidence-based health promotion program planning: perspective and examples. Front Public Health 2019;7:209.
18. Schmitzberger FF, Scott KW, Nham W, et al. Identifying strategies to boost COVID-19 vaccine acceptance in the United States. Rand Health Q 2022; 9(3):12.

19. Nowak GJ, Sheedy K, Bursey K, et al. Promoting influenza vaccination: insights from a qualitative meta-analysis of 14 years of influenza-related communications research by US Centers for Disease Control and Prevention (CDC). Vaccine 2015;33(24):2741–56.
20. Ning C, Guo D, Wu J, et al. Media exposure and media credibility influencing public intentions for influenza vaccination. Vaccines 2022;10(4):526.
21. Gollust SE, LoRusso SM, Nagler RH, et al. Understanding the role of the news media in HPV vaccine uptake in the United States: Synthesis and commentary. Hum Vaccin Immunother 2016;12(6):1430–4.
22. Borah P. Message framing and COVID-19 vaccination intention: Moderating roles of partisan media use and pre-attitudes about vaccination. Curr Psychol 2022. https://doi.org/10.1007/s12144-022-02851-3.
23. Jensen UT, Ayers S, Koskan AM. Video-based messages to reduce COVID-19 vaccine hesitancy and nudge vaccination intentions. PLoS One 2022;17(4): e0265736.
24. Crosby L, Rule A. Impact of COVID-19 on the LatinX and African-American Communities Paper presented at. CCTST Grand Rounds 2021; April;16:2021.
25. Marotta S, McNally VV. Increasing vaccine confidence through parent education and empowerment using clear and comprehensible communication. Acad Pediatr 2021;21(4):S30–1.
26. World Health Organization. Best practice guidance: how to respond to vocal vaccine deniers in public 2017. Available at: https://www.euro.who.int/__data/assets/pdf_file/0005/315761/Vocal-vaccine-deniers-guidance-document.pdf. Accessed June 1, 2022.
27. Streuli S, Ibrahim N, Mohamed A, et al. Development of a culturally and linguistically sensitive virtual reality educational platform to improve vaccine acceptance within a refugee population: the SHIFA community engagement-public health innovation programme. BMJ Open 2021;11(9):e051184.
28. Centers for Disease Control and Prevention. Vaccinate with Confidence. 2019. Available at: https://www.cdc.gov/vaccines/partners/vaccinate-with-confidence.html. Accessed June 1, 2022.
29. Dempsey AF, O'Leary ST. Human papillomavirus vaccination: Narrative review of studies on how providers' vaccine communication affects attitudes and uptake. Acad Pediatr 2018;18(2):S23–7.
30. Real FJ, DeBlasio D, Beck AF, et al. A virtual reality curriculum for pediatric residents decreases rates of influenza vaccine refusal. Acad Pediatr 2017;17(4): 431–5.
31. Gorstein A. giving childhood vaccinations a boost. 2019. 2022. Available at: https://www.ideas42.org/blog/giving-childhood-vaccinations-a-boost/.
32. Sims AM, Gomes SM, Crosby LE, et al. Partnering with Faith-based organizations to increase influenza vaccinations in children. Pediatrics 2022;150(3). e2022056193.
33. Schoeppe J, Cheadle A, Melton M, et al. The immunity community: a community engagement strategy for reducing vaccine hesitancy. Health Promotion Pract 2017;18(5):654–61.
34. Colorado Immunization Advocates. Colorado Immunization Advocates. 2017. Available at: http://www.coparents4vax.org/. Accessed June 14, 2022.
35. Leask J, Carlson SJ, Attwell K, et al. Communicating with patients and the public about COVID-19 vaccine safety: recommendations from the Collaboration on Social Science and Immunisation. Med J Aust 2021;215(1):9–12.

36. Sehgal NKR. Impact of vax-a-million lottery on COVID-19 vaccination rates in Ohio. Am J Med 2021;134(11):1424–6.
37. Campos-Mercade P, Meier AN, Schneider FH, et al. Monetary incentives increase COVID-19 vaccinations. Science 2021;374(6569):879–82.
38. Kim HB. Financial incentives for COVID-19 vaccination. Epidemiol Health 2021; 43:e2021088.
39. Wigham S, Ternent L, Bryant A, et al. Parental financial incentives for increasing preschool vaccination uptake: systematic review. Pediatrics 2014;134(4): e1117–28.
40. Smith LE, Hodson A, Rubin GJ. Parental attitudes towards mandatory vaccination; a systematic review. Vaccine 2021;39(30):4046–53.
41. Mulligan K, Harris JE. COVID-19 vaccination mandates for school and work are sound public policy. Available at: https://healthpolicy.usc.edu/wp-content/uploads/2022/07/USC_Schaeffer_Covid19-VaccineMandates_WhitePaper.pdf. Accessed August 1, 2022.
42. Greyson D, Vriesema-Magnuson C, Bettinger JA. Impact of school vaccination mandates on pediatric vaccination coverage: a systematic review. Can Med Assoc Open Access J 2019;7(3):E524–36.
43. Lee C, Robinson JL. Systematic review of the effect of immunization mandates on uptake of routine childhood immunizations. J Infect 2016;72(6):659–66.
44. Bardosh K, de Figueiredo A, Gur-Arie R, et al. The unintended consequences of COVID-19 vaccine policy: why mandates, passports and restrictions may cause more harm than good. BMJ Glob Health 2022;7(5):e008684.
45. Cataldi JR, Kerns ME, O'Leary ST. Evidence-based strategies to increase vaccination uptake: a review. Curr Opin Pediatr 2020;32(1):151–9.
46. Approved by the national vaccine advisory committee on september 17. 2020 national vaccine plan development: recommendations from the national vaccine advisory committee. Public Health Rep 2020;135(2):181–8.
47. El-Mohandes AA, Katz KS, El-Khorazaty MN, et al. The effect of a parenting education program on the use of preventive pediatric health care services among low-income, minority mothers: a randomized, controlled study. Pediatrics 2003; 111(6):1324–32.
48. Szilagyi PG, Schaffer S, Shone L, et al. Reducing geographic, racial, and ethnic disparities in childhood immunization rates by using reminder/recall interventions in urban primary care practices. Pediatrics 2002;110(5):e58.
49. Wood D, Halfon N, Donald-Sherbourne C, et al. Increasing immunization rates among inner-city, African American children: a randomized trial of case management. JAMA 1998;279(1):29–34.
50. Burkhardt MC, Real FJ, DeBlasio D, et al. Increasing coronavirus disease 2019 vaccine uptake in pediatric primary care by offering vaccine to household members. J Pediatr 2022;52(3):511–25.
51. Schaffer SJ, Rand CM, Humiston S, et al. Practical considerations in developing a successful school-located influenza vaccination (SLIV) program. Vaccine 2019; 37(16):2171–3.
52. Lindley MC, Boyer-Chu L, Fishbein DB, et al. The role of schools in strengthening delivery of new adolescent vaccinations. Pediatrics 2008;121(Supplement_1): S46–54.
53. Love H, Soleimanpour S, Panchal N, et al. National school-based health care census report. Paper presented at: School-Based Health Alliance 2018; April 16, 2021. Washington, DC.

54. Szilagyi PG, Schaffer S, Rand CM, et al. School-Located Influenza Vaccination: Do Vaccine Clinics at School Raise Vaccination Rates? J Sch Health 2019; 89(12):1004–12.
55. Kempe A, Allison MA, Daley MF. Can School-Located Vaccination Have a Major Impact on Human Papillomavirus Vaccination Rates in the United States? Acad Pediatr 2018;18(2, Supplement):S101–5.
56. Alden J, Crane K, robinson r, et al. Expansion of community pharmacies' role in public vaccine delivery to children: Opportunities and need. J Am Pharm Assoc 2022;62(5):1514–7.
57. Hess K, Bach A, Won K, et al. Community pharmacists roles during the COVID-19 pandemic. J Pharm Pract 2022;35(3):469–76.

9780443182303